The DOT Medical Examination

A Guide to Commercial Drivers' Medical Certification

Third Edition

Natalie P. Hartenbaum, MD, MPH

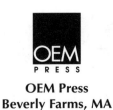

OEM Press
Beverly Farms, MA

ISBN: 1-883595-40-1

Printed in the United States of America

The recommendations contained in this book are based on reports sponsored by the Federal Highway Administration or other driver licensing agencies where available and should be used only as guidelines. They are not regulation unless specifically indicated as such. Sound medical knowledge and an understanding of the underlying disease process and progression must guide the final medical certification decision.

Library of Congress Cataloging in Publication data is available at http://cip.loc.gov/cip

OEM Press ® is a registered trademark of OEM Health Information, Inc.

Questions or comments regarding this book should be directed to:

OEM Health Information, Inc.
8 West Street
Beverly Farms, MA 01915-2226
978-921-7300
978-921-0304 (fax)
info@oempress.com

5   4

CONTENTS

CONTRIBUTING AUTHORS

Samuel D. Caughron, MD
Clinical Assistant Professor Family Practice
University of Virginia Medical School
Charlottesville, Virginia

Natalie P. Hartenbaum, MD, MPH
President and Chief Medical Officer
OccuMedix, Inc.
Dresher, Pennsylvania

Kurt T. Hegmann, MD, MPH
Research Associate Professor
Rocky Mountain Center for Occupational & Environmental Health
Department of Family and Preventive Medicine
University of Utah
Salt Lake City, Utah

Tuenis Zondag, MD, MPH
Occupational Medicine/Pain Medicine
Central Wyoming Neurosurgery
Casper, Wyoming

FOREWORD

Ensuring the medical fitness of the people who drive commercial motor vehicles is a challenge assumed by many physicians and other health professionals. Few would dispute the importance of promoting safety on our nation's highways, since the impact of accidents on people, property, and businesses can be devastating.

In follow-up to her first two successful editions, Dr. Natalie Hartenbaum, along with her contributors, has expanded the literature review on this national concern. The cardiac chapter includes the new guidelines from the Federal Motor Carrier cardiovascular advisory panel and there is an expanded chapter on the effects of medications on safe operations of commercial motor vehicles. After a historical overview of the history of the Federal Motor Carrier Safety Administration's effort at ensuring driver safety, the book then describes a model examination and current medical criteria used for evaluating work fitness. Specific organ systems, such a pulmonary and musculoskeletal, are addressed in full chapters, along with attention given to psychiatric disturbances and substance abuse, among others.

Natalie's book makes an important contribution to the practice of occupational medicine. By assembling disparate information from many sources, especially the Federal Register, this book provides a great service to practitioners by offering practical guidance in the conduct of commercial driver examinations. She appropriately emphasizes the importance of notifying the agency with suggestions for improving the quality of the process. In light of the fact that the physical qualifications have remained relatively unchanged over the past 30 years, such efforts should be applauded. Much has changed since 1970 — in medicine, especially in understanding the work implications of illnesses, and in laws, such as the enactment of The Americans with Disabilities Act. This book will help move the process forward in the development of medically sound and fair guidelines in assessing a person's ability to operate a commercial vehicle.

Robert J. McCunney, M.D., M.P.H.
Research Scientist, MIT, Department of Biological Engineering
Staff Physician, Massachusetts General Hospital
Harvard Medical School

PREFACE TO THE
THIRD EDITION

It is hard to believe that it's been six years since the first edition of this guide was published. We had hoped that this book would serve not only as a resource to occupational health professionals but also as a convenient reference for others involved in the commercial driver medical process. The extent to which this manual has been utilized has been beyond our imagination.

Much of the increased use of this book stems from the increasing attention that has been focused on the role that medical conditions may play in motor vehicle accidents. Several accident investigations by the National Transportation Safety Board (NTSB) have concluded that medical issues were a contributing cause. While much of the information has been available for years, it was not easily accessible nor were many examiners aware of its existence or location. Hopefully *The DOT Medical Examination; A Guide to Commercial Driver Medical Certification* had bridged that gap.

Since the second edition, there have been several changes in the medical certification process. The most significant has been the new examination reporting form that includes more information and guidance. Changes to the cardiac recommendation have been issued recently; and waiting for these to be available was the cause for the delay in publication date for this edition. There also will be updates to the form and the advisory criteria to reflect the new guidelines. Inconsistencies are noted and the reader is directed to the Chapter 4 for the most recent information. Also, while many chapters may reference the report from the Conference on Cardiac Disorders and Commercial Driver, the reader should refer to the Cardiovascular Advisory Panel Guidelines for the Medical Examination of Commercial Motor Vehicles Drivers[1] for the most updated information.

---

[1]Blumenthal R, Braunstein J, Connolly H, Epstein A, Gersh BJ, Wittels EH. *Cardiovascular Advisory Panel Guidelines for the Medical Examination of Commercial Motor Vehicle Drivers.* FMCSA-MCP-02-002. Washington: U.S. Department of Transportation, Federal Motor Carrier Safety Administration, October 2002.

While we stayed true to the original intent, compiling regulations and guidance in one easy-to-access place, we did expand the amount of recent medical literature review and provided comparisons with guidelines and regulations from countries that have reviewed and updated their stands more recently than the United States.

Once again, I want to thank Drs. Sam Caughron, Kurt Hegmann, and Tuenis Zondag, who put up with my changes in format, editing and pestering to meet deadlines. Sandra Zywokarte, Acting Chief, Physical Qualifications Division of the Federal Motor Carrier Safety Administration continues to be a great resource and I know her assistance is appreciated by the medical examiner community. A thanks also to Dr. Mitch Garber, Medical Officer of the NTSB for his assistance in identification of accidents where medical conditions were implicated. The support and encouragement by Curtis Vouwie of OEM Press continues to be invaluable.

And last but not least, special thanks to my husband Dave, who continues to encourage and stand beside me in my continually evolving projects. And to Sara and Alissa, who get excited seeing their name in a book, their excitement, enthusiasm and love, make everything worthwhile.

We all hope this third edition meets your expectations and needs.

NATALIE P. HARTENBAUM, MD, MPH

I

The Examination Process

1

Commercial Driver Medical Qualification: Past, Present, and Future

NATALIE P. HARTENBAUM, MD, MPH

Health care professionals who examine commercial drivers to determine medical fitness often comment that the regulations are old and out of step with current knowledge. While this may be true, the current standard is a significant improvement over the initial criteria from June 7, 1939, requiring the following minimum qualifications: "Good physical and mental health; good eyesight; adequate hearing; no addiction to narcotic drugs; and no excessive use of alcoholic beverages or liquors" [1].

The Motor Carrier Safety Act of 1935 granted the Interstate Commerce Commission (ICC) the authority to require medical certification for operators of commercial motor vehicles (CMVs) but not physical examinations. A physical examination and Certificate of Physical Evaluation were not required until January 1, 1954.

The U.S. Department of Transportation (DOT) was created by an act of Congress in 1970. Responsibility for commercial driver qualification was transferred to the DOT the same year. Tighter medical qualification standards were announced 30 years to the day after issuance of the initial criteria, on June 7, 1969 [2].

Physical requirements at that time were similar to those of the current standard. In the original notice, insulin use in the 12 months preceding the examination was disqualifying, as was a blood pressure above 160/90 mm Hg. The audiometric criterion in the Notice of Proposed Rulemaking was an average loss not greater than 25 to 30 dB in the better ear. Examinations were proposed to be required annually. However, in the Final Rule, issued on April 22, 1970 [3], the frequency of the examination was changed to biennial. The blood pressure criterion also was changed to its current form, disqualifying only those whose elevated blood pressure was "likely to interfere with the driver's ability to safely operate a commercial motor vehicle." The Final Rule also stated that only current use of insulin would be considered cause for disqualification. The use of hearing aids to meet the audiometric standard became permissible in 1971. At the same time, the maximal permissible hearing loss was increased to an average loss not greater than 40 dB in the better ear. Since 1971, the physical qualification standards have remained essentially unchanged.

Over the years, there have been several changes to the medical examination process. When controlled substance testing was initially implemented, testing was part of the periodic medical fitness examination. Once a company was conducting random tests at a 50 percent annual rate, periodic controlled substance testing could be discontinued. In July 1997, reference to subpart H, drug testing, was formally eliminated, and any reference to drug testing as part of the physical examination was removed [4]. Now that random testing is fully in effect, the only situation where the drug test and the examination might be done at the same office visit is in a preplacement situation. Even in this circumstance, the medical evaluation and the drug test should be considered as two separate and unrelated processes.

A 1992 amendment to the Federal Motor Carrier Safety Regulations (FMCSRs) allowed licensed health care professionals other than physicians to perform the examinations [5]. Some physician assistants, advanced practice nurses under physician supervision, and doctors of chiropractic are now able to evaluate commercial drivers for qualification. These providers can perform commercial driver medical examinations only if the state in which they are licensed permits them to perform such examinations. The hope was that by expanding the examiner pool there would be greater flexibility in arranging the required examination and possibly lower cost.

As a result of the Americans with Disabilities Act, the Congress directed the Federal Highway Administration (FHWA) to perform a thorough review of the physical qualifications. Announcements that studies were proposed to consider the feasibility of relaxing the vision [6] and diabetes [7] standards were published in the *Federal Register* in 1992 and 1993, respectively. The diabetes waiver program would permit some drivers with at least a 3-year record of safe commercial vehicle driving to drive a CMV in interstate commerce. Several other conditions were set, including blood sugar monitoring and the reporting of any accident, whether or not it normally would have been reportable. Some commercial drivers with at least a 3-year safe driving record and at least 20/40 vision corrected or uncorrected in the better eye were eligible for the vision waiver program.

A suit filed by the Advocates for Highway and Auto Safety requested a review of the issuance of waivers to individuals who otherwise did not meet the federal standard. In 1994, the U.S. Court of Appeals for the D.C. Circuit found that the "agency's determination that the waiver program(s) will not adversely affect the safe operation of CMVs is devoid of empirical support" [8]. New applications for these waiver programs are not currently being accepted, but those drivers currently holding waivers were grandfathered to continue to operate in interstate commerce provided they continue to meet requirements [9–10]. A hearing waiver program to review the hearing standard was proposed in 1993 but was never begun [11].

A 1996 Eighth Circuit Court decision, in *Rauenhorst v. United States Department of Transportation*, required the agency to consider granting a waiver to a driver who met the criteria for a waiver prior to the program being closed [12]. Since this decision, a number of drivers, initially in the area covered by the jurisdiction of the Eighth Circuit Court, have been granted waivers and more recently exemptions. Formal procedures for waivers, exemptions, and pilot programs were announced in 1998 [13]. Waivers and exemptions are temporary relief from one or more of the FMCSRs. Waivers are valid for up to 3 months, whereas exemptions may be valid for up to 2 years and are renewable. For both, the applicant must indicate how the same or a greater level of safety could be achieved if the relief were granted. An exemption decision requires an opportunity for public comment, through publication in the *Federal Register*, whereas waivers do not. The only exemption to the medical standards that is currently being considered is for those drivers not meeting the vision standard.

A 2000 report to Congress [14] on the feasibility of qualifying individuals with insulin-treated diabetes reviewed the issue and offered suggestions on how to permit some drivers on insulin to operate commercial vehicles in interstate commerce. There is consideration to grant exemptions to drivers who require insulin for control of their diabetes. A Request for Comments was published in the July 31, 2001, *Federal Register* [15]. The comment period closed October 2001, and there have been no further announcements.

Drivers who have been unable to meet the first or second medical standard because of a loss or impairment of an extremity had been eligible for a limb waiver. In May 2000 [16], terminology for this variance from the standards was changed to refer to a Skill Performance Evaluation (SPE) certificate rather than a waiver. This is now signed by the Division Administrator of the FMCSA. A road test is also required prior to issuance of the SPE.

A negotiated rule-making committee was formed in 1996 [17] and charged with identifying a method for merging the commercial driver's license process with the medical qualification process. The need to improve the quality of examinations was particularly significant. "Doctor shopping" and the lack of understanding by many examiners of the regulations and supporting material were identified as a significant problem. Several proposals were discussed to enhance consistency among health care providers performing commercial driver medical examinations. The proposals ranged from requiring examiners to sign a statement indicating that they understand the regulations and agree to follow them to an extensive certification course. The final meeting of the committee occurred in November 1997, and publication of the proposed rule making is still pending. A likely method may require a health care provider, who, by virtue of his or her professional license, could perform these examinations, to apply to a national registry. An information packet containing the standards, regulatory criteria, and other guidance material would be provided. A database of approved providers would permit distribution of updates to the standards, procedures, or regulatory criteria as they become available.

Motor carrier safety had been under the authority of the FHWA until October 1999, when responsibility was transferred to the Federal Motor Carrier Safety Administration (FMCSA) which reports directly to the secretary of the DOT [18].

Consistent with the definitions used in the Transportation Equity Act for the Twenty-first Century (TEA-21), the FHWA amended the definition of a commercial vehicle under 390.5, which is used for determining which vehicles are subject to the FMCSRs, including the medical standards [19]. The definition also now includes vehicles designed or used to carry more than eight passengers (including the driver) for compensation. In the same announcement, the FHWA delayed requiring operators of smaller vehicles to comply with these regulations until at least March 6, 2000. The FHWA reported that there were no data to demonstrate that changing the requirements would improve safety. Therefore, operators of smaller vehicles would be exempt while further study is undertaken. On January 11, 2001, a Notice of Proposed Rulemaking requested comments on requiring operators of vehicles designed to carry eight to fifteen passengers, including the driver, to comply with hours of service requirements and to obtain medical certification examinations [20]. While the comment period closed in April 2001, a Final Rule has not been published. In 2001, an Advanced Notice of Proposed Rulemaking was published [21], requesting comments on possibly requiring school bus drivers involved in interstate transport of students (excluding home to school and return) to comply with the FMCSRs, including a medical examination. The comment period closed in January 2002, and no further announcements have been published.

One of the most significant changes in the medical certification process was the development and implementation of a new form. The proposed new form was published in the *Federal Register* in 1998 [22], and the Final Rule was published on October 5, 2000 [23]. This form includes one page each for medical history, testing, and recording of the physical examination. Instructions to examiners, the role of the commercial driver, and inclusion of the advisory criteria bring the entire document to eight pages. The advisory criteria reference the conference reports and provide phone numbers for additional questions on issues such as Coumadin use. The examiner is also advised that additional information, either from the treating provider or a specialist, may be necessary. The option to certify a driver for less than 24 months if a medical condition is present that does not disqualify, but would require more frequent monitoring, is clearly stated. The examiner is directed to sign the certificate only if the driver would be able to perform both driving *and* nondriving duties.

Drivers are instructed to complete the history segment and then sign a statement indicating that the history they provided is accurate. The medical history questions are more relevant, and there is a place to list any medication the driver is taking. In addition, questions on venereal disease and the place for recording serology are no longer included. The examiner is instructed to review medication, and a question on sleep disorders has been added. The testing and physical examination pages include many of the standards adjacent to where the examiner would enter findings, e.g., vision or blood pressure. Pulse after exercise is no longer required.

With the document including not just the history and physical examination but also some guidance material, it was anticipated that examiners would have and utilize the necessary information. In their 1998 report on a New Orleans bus accident [24], the National Transportation Safety Board (NTSB) identified the failure of the medical certification program to detect the driver's medical problems and remove him from service as one of the probable causes of the accident. The NTSB believed that the new form was a substantial improvement in serving as a resource for the medical examiner.

Neither the form nor the certificate included in the October 5, 2000, *Federal Register* must be used exactly as published. Forms and certificates used must be "substantially in accordance" with the published versions. The examination reporting form can be reformatted or completed electronically. The certificate (commonly referred to as the card) can be resized to fit into a wallet and is not required to be any specific paper stock weight.

New guidelines and regulations will continue to be issued. As examiners, it is important that we stay abreast of new developments and studies. Watch for *Federal Register* announcements that affect the medical qualification process. Write to the FMCSA voicing your support, opinions, or concerns regarding proposals. Keep track of situations where you feel the regulations are inadequate or where inconsistencies exist. Also note cases where a driver has "doctor shopped" and been certified despite not meeting criteria. Above all, be certain that the examinations you provide are within regulations and guidelines and based on current medical knowledge.

As this is rushing to press, new Cardiovascular Guidelines have become available. They are reviewed in Chapter 4.

References

1. Zywokarte S. Team Leader, Driver Medical Standards, FHWA. Personal communication, October 1996.
2. Qualification of drivers. *Fed Reg* 1969;34(June 7):9080–9085.
3. Qualification of drivers of commercial motor vehicles. *Fed Reg* 1970;35(April 22):6458–6467.
4. Commercial driver's license program and controlled substances and alcohol use and testing: Conforming and technical amendments. *Fed Reg* 1997;62(July 11):37150–37153.
5. Qualification of drivers: Medical examination. *Fed Reg* 1992;57(July 28):33276.
6. Qualification of drivers: Waiver applications—vision. *Fed Reg* 1992;57(March 25):10295–10297.
7. Qualification of drivers: Waivers—diabetes. *Fed Reg* 1993;58(July 29):40690–40697.
8. Qualification of drivers: Vision deficiencies—waivers. *Fed Reg* 1994;59(Nov. 17):39386–39390.
9. Qualification of drivers: Vision and diabetes—limited exemptions. *Fed Reg* 1996;61(Jan. 8):606–611.
10. Qualification of drivers: Vision and diabetes—limited exemptions. *Fed Reg* 1996;61(March 26):13338–13347.
11. Qualification of drivers: Hearing deficiencies—waivers. *Fed Reg* 1993;58(Dec. 15):65638–65643.

12. Qualification of drivers: Waiver application—vision. *Fed Reg* 1998;63(Jan. 8):1524–1537.
13. Federal Motor Carrier Safety Regulations: Waivers, exemptions, and pilot programs—rules and procedures. *Fed Reg* 1998;63(Dec. 8):67600–67612.
14. A Report to Congress on the Feasibility of a Program to Qualify Individuals with Insulin Treated Diabetes Mellitus to Operate Commercial Motor Vehicles in Interstate Commerce as Directed by the Transportation Equity Act for the 21st Century. July 2000.
15. Notice of intent to issue exemptions and request for comments; Qualification of Drivers; Exemption applications; Diabetes. *Fed Reg* 2001;66(July 31):39548–39553.
16. Federal Motor Carrier Safety Regulations; Technical amendments; Final rule; Technical amendment. *Fed Reg* 2000;65(May 1):25285–25290.
17. Commercial driver physical qualifications as a part of the commercial driver's license process. *Fed Reg* 1996;61(April 29):18713–18717.
18. Organization and delegation of powers and duties: Redelegation to the director, Office of Motor Carrier Safety. *Fed Reg* 1999;64(Oct. 29):56270–56271.
19. Federal Motor Carrier Safety Regulations: Definitions of commercial motor vehicle—interim final rule; Federal Motor Carrier Safety Regulations: Requirements for operators of small passenger-carrying commercial motor vehicles—proposed rule. *Fed Reg* 1999;64(Sept. 3):48510–48517.
20. Safety requirements for operators of small passenger-carrying commercial motor vehicles used in interstate commerce; Notice of proposed rulemaking; Request for comments. *Fed Reg* 2001;66(Jan. 11);2767–2779.
21. Interstate school bus safety; Advanced notice of proposed rulemaking; Request for comments. *Fed Reg* 2001;66(Oct. 22):53373–53376.
22. Physical qualification of drivers: Medical examination—certificate. *Fed Reg* 1998;63(Aug. 5):41769–41781.
23. Physical qualification of drivers; Medical examination; Final rule. *Fed Reg* 2000;65(Oct. 5):59363–59380.
24. National Transportation Safety Board. Highway Accident Report: Motorcoach Run-Off-The-Road. New Orleans, Louisiana, May 9, 1999: HAR-01-01, 08/28/2001 NTIS Report No. PB2001–916201.

2

Commercial Driver Medical Certification—The Examination

Tuenis Zondag, MD

Since the previous edition of this book, the Federal Motor Carrier Safety Administration (FMCSA) has implemented the use of a new medical examination form. This form is easier to follow and contains a significant amount of guidance material. The change was intended "to gain simplicity and efficiency, to reflect current medical terminology and examination components, and to be a self-contained document (the form will, to the extent possible, include all relevant information necessary to conduct the physical examination and certification)" [1]. The new form also requires the driver to sign that the "information is accurate and complete and that inaccurate, false, or missing information may invalidate both the examination and any medical examination certification issued based upon it" [1]. While the advisory criteria were updated with the new form, the physical qualification standards used by medical examiners have not been changed.

The medical examiner is expected to use sound medical judgment in determining whether an individual is medically qualified to operate a commercial motor vehicle (CMV). The medical standards are codified and have a statutory basis. The FMCSA provides additional guidance for the examiner to use. These recommendations, called advisory criteria, are intended to help the examiner determine whether the driver meets the physical standards. These are included on the new form. Additional guidance is available in the form of reports from conferences sponsored by the Federal Highway Administration (FHWA) [2–5]. Many of these publications can be found on the FMCSA Internet site at *http://www.fmcsa.dot.gov/rulesregs/medreports.htm*.

Other countries have developed published recommendations for CMV drivers [6–7]. FMCSA medical examinations may be performed by physicians (MD or DO), physician assistants, advanced practice nurses, or chiropractors, depending on state licensure or registration.

10

The medical examiner must be aware of the physical, mental, and social demands placed on the CMV driver, as well as the regulations [1]. The new FMCSA medical form includes information on both the physical qualification standards and tests required to assess whether the driver meets these standards. The CMV driver must meet the minimum medical standards and must be able to perform both driving and nondriving duties before the examiner should sign the medical certificate and form. "The FMCSA's primary concern is to enhance highway safety, not to necessarily limit employment opportunities for individuals with physical handicaps" [1]. In the interest of public safety, the medical examiner is required to certify that the driver does not have any physical, mental, or organic conditions that might affect the driver's ability to operate a CMV safely" [1].

For the purpose of the medical examination, a CMV is defined by 49 CFR 390.5 as follows:

"Commercial motor vehicle (CMV) means any self-propelled or towed vehicle used on public highways in interstate commerce to transport passengers or property when:

(a) The vehicle has a gross weight rating or gross combination of 10,001 pounds or more; or

(b) The vehicle is designed or used to transport more than 8 passengers (including the driver) for compensation; or

(c) Is designed or used to transport more than 15 passengers, including the driver, and is not used to transport passengers for compensation; or

(d) Is used in the transporting of materials found by the Secretary of Transportation to be hazardous under 49 CFR U.S.C. 5103 and transporting in a quantity requiring placarding under regulations prescribed by the Secretary under 49 CFR, subtitle B, chapter I, subchapter C."

While Rulemaking is in progress, vehicles designed to transport eight to fifteen passengers, including the driver, do not require a physical examination at this time.

If an impairment or medical condition is identified during the examination, the examiner should consider whether the individual's impairment(s) will affect the ability to operate a CMV safely. The medical determination should be based on the history, physical examination, and, if needed, additional medical information that the medical examiner believes is necessary to arrive at a decision. The examiner must determine whether the medical condition will remain stable or may deteriorate over the certification period. Particular attention must also be paid to the risks and benefits a medication may have on a CMV driver and his or her performance of duties in all potential work situations.

In many cases where the driver has existing medical conditions, additional medical information or specialist evaluations may be required. The examiner should obtain the driver's written permission. Prior to requesting any additional information or examination, the party responsible for any additional costs, whether the employer or the employee, should be identified.

Based upon an unpublished survey of commercial drivers, the commercial drivers were found to have health or demographic characteristics that placed them at high risk to develop medical conditions [8]. These conditions included elevated blood pressure or early hypertension; poor control of diabetes or abnormal screening blood sugars; higher levels of obesity (body mass index [BMI] > 30); higher prevalence of smoking than the general public (approximately 47 percent); multiple musculoskeletal impairments; cardiac, pulmonary, and neurologic impairments; and medications used for pain control, psychiatric conditions, and cardiac, pulmonary, diabetic, and weight loss disorders.

The new medical forms require about 10 to 20 minutes to complete. The examiner is expected to comment on any "Yes" answer in the medical history and the effect upon the CMV operation. Any "Yes" checked on the physical examination form must also have a comment upon its effect upon the CMV operation. Based on the unpublished survey and personal experience, about one in three drivers were given less than a 2-year certification, as they had medical conditions that did not prohibit driving but required closer monitoring [8]. The new medical examination form contains an option for the examiner to have the driver return for additional evaluation. The examiner may complete the statement for the driver to "Return to medical examiner's office for follow-up on _____."

When a CMV driver or candidate presents for an examination, this author's staff measures the height, weight, blood pressure, pulse, vision, and hearing and tests the urine for glucose, blood, and protein. The examiner must review these and make sure the entire form is completed. My experience is that many drivers are guarded, and an attitude of caring helps to improve the process. The entire interview performed by both the staff and the examiner should be used to assess emotional stability. It is important to review the questions on cardiac function, pulmonary function, fatigue, sleep habits, medications, and musculoskeletal function in Part II before moving on to the other sections.

There are four absolute codified criteria that must be met. If the driver does not meet any of these, he or she should be disqualified. These four criteria are:

1. Vision must be at least 20/40 in both eyes, with or without correction; peripheral vision must be ≥ 70 degrees in the horizontal plane; and the driver must be able to identify colors of traffic signals (red, green, and amber). (Some drivers who do not have vision correctable to at least 20/40 in either eye may be eligible for an exemption.)

2. The driver cannot have an average hearing loss at 500, 1000, and 2000 Hz >40 dB in the better ear. This is calculated by adding the value at 500, 1000, and 2000 Hz in one ear and dividing by three. A hearing aid can be used to meet the criteria.

3. The driver cannot have a clinical diagnosis of diabetes mellitus requiring insulin for control.

4. Established medical history of epilepsy or clinical diagnosis of epilepsy is disqualifying. This would include the use of antiseizure medications.

While the use of methadone is not codified as an absolute disqualification, it is explained in both advisory criteria and Regulatory Guidance that a commercial driver should not be qualified if on methadone [9].

The examiner must be aware of the job functions, work environment, and work schedule based on information from the "The Driver's Role," as described on the examination form.

The remaining part of the examination should be used to address the following areas:

1. *General Appearance:* Consider assessing for sleep disorders when the following three risk factors are present: weight > 70 percent normal, hypertension, and neck size > 17 inches [10]. Tremor, abnormal finger-to-nose test, and abnormal balance may be associated with neurologic abnormalities.

2. *Eyes:* Measure visual acuity, horizontal field of vision, and the ability to recognize red, green, and amber (many individuals

with color vision deficiency are able to identify the colors of the signal). Remember to check boxes for monocular vision. If the driver does not meet the vision criteria, he or she should not be qualified until an exemption has been obtained. Evaluate the mobility of each eye, up/down/left/right lateral motions. I perform a fundoscopic examination if a medical condition associated with retinal disease is known. If abnormalities are found, record them and comment whether they would affect the operation of a CMV safely.

3. *Ears:* Screen for hearing abnormalities in each ear. If found, perform a booth audiogram for hearing loss at 500, 1000, and 2000 Hz. Drivers with an average hearing loss of >40 dB (with or without hearing aids) do not meet the medical standard. Inspection of the canal and tympanic membrane is an important part of the examination.

4. *Mouth and Throat:* Evaluate for conditions of lip, tongue, and pharynx that produce conditions likely to interfere with breathing, speaking, or swallowing.

5. *Neck:* The neck must have mobility to see the gauges forward, upward, and the mirrors to the left and right. Critical neck mobility may vary from vehicle to vehicle. This examiner found the critical range of motion (directly measured with a goniometer in a late-model 1990 Freight Liner Conventional truck) to be 30 degrees rotation to the left, 45 degrees rotation to the right, 40 degrees flexion downward, and 20 degrees flexion upward.

6. *Heart:* The cardiac area should be assessed by inspection (incisions from surgery), palpation (heart lift or thrill), and auscultation (murmurs and extra sounds). It is important to assess whether an individual may have inadvertently missed commenting on a history of cardiac disease or surgery. If abnormalities are found, one must assess for the potential of cardiac ischemia or the risk of syncope or congestive heart failure. If the driver has a history of cardiac disease, the examiner should request old medical records or indicate recommended additional assessment.

7. *Blood Pressure/Pulse Rate:* There are very specific guidelines in the new form (Section 5). They will be updated to be consistent with new guidelines (see Chapter 4).

8. *Lung and Chest (not to include breast exam):* Sufficient pulmonary function is required. The examiner's inspection (abnormal

expansion and incisions) and auscultation (abnormal sounds) allows for a medical decision as to whether an individual has respiratory dysfunction. An approach to making the judgment can be obtained from the conference on pulmonary/respiratory disorders and the commercial driver [5] or in the Pulmonary Disorders chapter of this book.

9. *Abdomen and Viscera:* Inspection, auscultation, and palpation should be used to assess the abdominal contents. CMV drivers with findings of enlarged liver, spleen, masses, or abdominal bruits need further medical assessment to determine whether illness is present that would interfere with safe CMV driving. Hernias and abdominal wall weaknesses may be found on examination, and the examiner must determine whether this may interfere with driving. Although there is no good reference for disqualification, this examiner finds large inguinal hernias, abdominal hernias, and significant abdominal wall loss and weakness to be grounds to assess whether an individual can perform the essentials of the job the company requires for safe job functioning besides driving.

10. *Vascular System:* Inspection of the lower extremities for large varicosities and skin abnormalities and edema is expected. Carotids should be assessed for pulses and bruits. If abnormal circulation in the arterial system, central nervous system, or peripheral limbs is found, the examiner should determine whether a more detailed evaluation is required or whether the driver meets the medical criteria but should be certified for a shorter period of time. Adequate lower extremity function is necessary to ensure safe operation of these vehicles.

11. *Extremities:* Good functioning of upper and lower extremities is critical to safe motor vehicle operation. If an examiner finds abnormal function in any upper or lower extremity either by loss of limb or other impairment, the driver does not meet the criteria but may be eligible for a Skill Performance Evaluation Certificate. Based on this examiner's observations of requirement for safe cab entrance (cab-overs or conventional cabs) and exit, a shoulder mobility right and left of 120 degrees is critical (measured with a goniometer). This examiner uses as his guideline the following handgrip recommendation. This recommendation is based on regular handgrip measurement done as part of the FMCSA examination I did over a number of years and successful driving by all drivers evaluated. The driver should have a good handgrip (equivalent to the average female

handgrip of 24.6 kg or 54.1 lb) to handle a vehicle with or without power drive [11]. The driver must have good wrist power to operate a vehicle based on an examination of finger curling and flexion of the wrist against resistance (gripping and turning the steering wheel) [12]. My approach to drivers with weakness observed is to have the safety officer of the company hiring do a road test. Failure to perform safely leads me to disqualify these individuals. Many driving situations require different critical function levels to operate the CMV safely. Lower extremity evaluation by FABER maneuver (flexion of the hip with abduction and external rotation), significant limp, significant ankle rigidity, and significant reduction in foot plantar flexion (reduced ability to step on brakes and accelerators) can lead one to require an observed drive by the proposed company safety officer to determine safe handling of the vehicle.

12. *Spine:* The spine is the major support structure of the body. It is important to inspect for surgical scars, deformities (kyphosis, scoliosis), loss of range of motion, and evidence of painful motion. This examiner uses as his guideline (based on a 45-degree bend or stoop) observation of drivers inspecting trailers (flatbed and reefers). The driver's back function depends upon job function and may require loading/unloading, tie downs, tarping, and pulling down of hoses. The driver must tolerate different positions: sitting, bending to inspect, climbing, squatting, and pushing or pulling such as fifth wheel pins. Back disorders, according to the unpublished survey, are common to CMV drivers, and any abnormality and/or restriction should be considered in relationship to the job function when certifying.

13. *Neurologic:* This system is critical to proper job functioning. Assessment of gait, equilibrium, command of language through interview, and reflexes in the upper and lower extremities for symmetry are methods that should be used to evaluate this system. If significant abnormalities are found, further medical evaluation may be required before qualification status can be determined. Drivers should have sufficient language and speech skills to carry on simple conversations and understand moderate levels of instruction, such as finding new drop locations from listening or computer reading. These requirements are job critical skill functions, and if not present, disqualification should be considered unless accommodated in an alternate manner.

14. *Laboratory and Other Test Findings:* Urinalysis is required. This examiner evaluates any level of glucosuria with a random blood

sugar. See the Endocrine Disorders chapter in this book for an approach. If significant proteinuria or hematuria is found, the driver should be informed and instructed to follow-up with his or her personal physician. The examiner should determine whether the abnormalities represent a problem that may make the driver unsafe or whether a shorter certification period would be appropriate.

15. *GYN and Rectal Examinations:* These examinations are not required for CMV driver's certification.

16. *Mental Status:* Although not on the form, 49 CFR 391.41, Part 9, requires that the driver "has no mental, nervous, organic, or functional disease, or psychiatric disorder likely to interfere with his ability to drive a commercial motor vehicle safely." This area of functioning can be assessed by the driver's cooperative nature during the entire exam, by the flow of information on questioning, and by the driver's attitude. Excessive antagonism, aggressiveness, abnormal sexual overtones, paranoia, or severe depression should cause the examiner to evaluate the driver more carefully. This examiner has, on occasion, temporarily disqualified an individual and required additional evaluation at the driver's expense. When this examiner encounters such drivers, they are evaluated annually for an indefinite period. Information from their personal physician is required as to whether they feel this driver can safely operate a CMV. Emotional instability and personality disorders may warrant disqualification.

In the new form, the driver's role has been well delineated. The CMV driver with a larger than normal vehicle must use appropriate perceptual skills to monitor a sometimes complex driving situation. Drivers must use appropriate judgment skills to make quick decisions and manipulative skills to control the vehicle. They must be able to drive safely and defensively in all types of weather and motoring conditions. Additionally, their job functions may include coupling and uncoupling trailers, loading and unloading trailers, placing and removing tarpaulins, tying down equipment or materials, and pushing or pulling hoses from a tanker. The examiner is required to assess the driver to see that the individual can safely perform the essentials of the job, including the work besides driving.

Before the examiner or office staff starts the medical examination, certain information must be known. Who is responsible for the cost of the examination, testing, and procedures (e.g., blood test, electrocardiogram, x-rays) if required? The examiner and/or staff should use the driver's photo identification to ensure that the appropriate person is examined. The new driver's medical examination card must be marked with the practitioner's name, state and medical license number, and office address and phone number. Ideally, this is either printed or stamped so that the information is legible. The medical certification expiration is now on the card, as well as the date of the examination.

This author found in his unpublished survey that one of three drivers received less than a 2-year certification based upon medical judgment. The new form requires the examiner to explain further all the "Yes" responses and how they affect medical certification to drive or perform essential job functions. Most CMV drivers live a lifestyle that places them at risk for fatigue, sleep problems, and medical problems. It is the examiner's job to assess whether the CMV driver meets the minimum standards to drive and safely inspect, manipulate, operate, and perform the essentials of that driver's job function.

References

1. Physical qualification of drivers; Medical examination; Certification. *Fed Reg* 2000;65(Oct. 5):59363–59380.
2. U.S. Department of Transportation, Federal Highway Administration. *Conference on Cardiac Disorders and the Commercial Driver.* Publication No. FHWA-MC-88-040. Washington: U.S. DOT, Federal Highway Administration, Office of Motor Carriers, 1987.
3. U.S. Department of Transportation, Federal Highway Administration. *Conference on Neurological Disorders and the Commercial Driver.* Publication No. FHWA-MC-88-042. Washington: U.S. DOT, Federal Highway Administration, Office of Motor Carriers, 1988.
4. U.S. Department of Transportation, Federal Highway Administration. *Conference on Psychiatric Disorders and the Commercial Driver.* Publication No. FHWA-MC-91-006. Washington: U.S. DOT, Federal Highway Administration, Office of Motor Carriers, 1990.
5. U.S. Department of Transportation, Federal Highway Administration. *Conference on Pulmonary/Respiratory Disorders and the Commercial Driver.* Publication No. FHWA-MC-91-004. Washington: U.S. DOT, Federal Highway Administration, Office of Motor Carriers, 1991.
6. Driver and Vehicle Licensing Agency. *At-a-Glance Guide to the Current Medical Standards of Fitness to Drive.* Swansea, England: Drivers

Medical Unit, DVLA, 2002. *http:www.dula.gov.uk/at_a_glance/ content.html.* Accessed Oct. 6, 2002.

7. Australian Faculty of Occupational Medicine. *Medical Examinations of Commercial Vehicle Drivers.* Prepared for the National Road Transport Commission and the Federal Office of Road Safety. *http://www.nrtc.gov.au/publications/med-stand.asp?lo=public.* Accessed Oct. 6, 2002.

8. Zondag T. *Length of Certification of Commercial Drivers.* Unpublished study.

9. Regulatory Guidance for the Federal Motor Safety Regulation; Rules. Section 394.41. Physical Qualifications for Drivers, Question 4. *Fed Reg* 1997;62(April 4):16369–16431. *http://www.fmcsa.dot.gov/ rulesregs/fmcsr/final/040497.txt.* Accessed Oct. 6, 2002.

10. U.S. Department of Transportation, Federal Motor Carrier Safety Administration. *Effects of Sleep Schedules on Commercial Motor Vehicle Driver Performance.* Report No. DOT-MC-00-133. Washington: Federal Motor Carrier Safety Administration, 2000.

11. Swanson AB, Matev IB, deGroot G. The strength of the hand. *Bull Prosthet Res* Fall 1970:145–153.

12. Roberts WN, Roberts PC. Evaluation of the elderly driver with arthritis. *Clin Geriatr Med* 1993;9(2):311–322.

Additional References

Pommerenke F, Hegmann K, Hartenbaum NP. DOT examinations: Practical aspects and regulatory review. *Am Fam Phys* 1998;58(2):415–426.

Wells JL, Ferreira DC. Guidelines for the Department of Transportation physical examination. *Nurse Pract* 1999;24(5):78, 81, 88–92.

3

Regulations, Advisory Criteria, and Regulatory Guidance

NATALIE P. HARTENBAUM, MD, MPH

Many examiners thought that the only information they needed to perform the commercial driver medical examination was provided on the old form. Whereas the old form, which had been in use until 2001, contained only the medical standards and instructions to examiners, the new form also includes the advisory criteria. Although this new form can be considered to be self-contained, there are still many other parts of the Federal Motor Carrier Safety Regulations (FMCSRs) that the examiner should be aware of prior to signing the medical certificate. These other parts indicate whether the driver is qualified in accordance with 49 CFR 391.41 through 391.49, yet many examiners are not aware that only 391.41 is covered entirely on the form. This chapter includes most of the regulations relevant to the commercial driver medical certification program. For those accustomed to the advisory criteria being separate, they are now included on the form. The Regulatory Guidance related to those regulations is also included in this chapter. The Regulatory Guidance consists of responses to specific questions and was most recently published in the Federal Register on April 4, 1997. Periodic updates as well as all the Regulations, complete Regulatory Guidance, Rulemaking Announcements, and Medical Conference Reports can be accessed through the Federal Motor Carrier Safety Administration's Internet site (http://www.fmcsa.dot.gov).

The entire medical examination is included in this chapter. Portions of the final five pages of the form, including driver roles, instructions to examiners, and advisory criteria, have been reproduced for easier reading. The only section not reproduced is the standards themselves, 391.41, as they are listed in both the full text of the regulations and the advisory criteria.

Note that the weight used to define a commercial vehicle in 49 CFR 390.5 (FMCSRs, which includes the medical requirements) differs from that found in 49 CFR 382 (Controlled Substances and Alcohol Use and Testing) and 383 (Commercial Driver's License). In the sections on controlled substance testing and commercial driver's license, a commercial motor vehicle is defined as a motor vehicle or combination of motor vehicles used in commerce to transport passengers or property if the motor vehicle

1. Has a gross combination weight rating of 11,794 kg or more (26,001 lb or more) inclusive of a towed unit with a gross vehicle weight rating of more than 4536 kg (10,000 lb); or

2. Has a gross vehicle weight rating of 11,794 kg or more (26,001 lb or more); or

3. Is designed to transport sixteen or more passengers, including the driver; or

4. Is of any size and is used in the transportation of materials found to be hazardous for the purposes of the Hazardous Materials Transportation Act and that require the motor vehicle to be placarded under the Hazardous Materials Regulations (49 CFR part 172, subpart F).

To determine which drivers fall under the FMCSRs regarding medical examination, in addition to operators of vehicles that transport hazardous material requiring placarding, the following weights and passenger capacities are used:

1. Has a gross vehicle weight rating or gross combination weight rating, or gross vehicle weight or gross combination weight, of 4537 kg (10,001 lb) or more, whichever is greater; or

2. Is designed or used to transport more than eight passengers (including the driver) for compensation; or

3. Is designed or used to transport more than fifteen passengers

Whether operators of vehicles designed to carry eight to fifteen passengers for direct compensation will be required to meet the medical standards has not been determined. A January 11, 2001, Federal Register announcement proposed that they would, but a final rule has not yet been published.

Selected section from
TITLE 49—TRANSPORTATION

CHAPTER III—FEDERAL MOTOR CARRIER SAFETY ADMINISTRATION, DEPARTMENT OF TRANSPORTATION

§390.5   Definitions—only those pertaining to examination are included—The complete section 390.5 can be found through the FMCSA webpage.

Commercial motor vehicle means any self-propelled or towed motor vehicle used on a highway in interstate commerce to transport passengers or property when the vehicle

(1) Has a gross vehicle weight rating or gross combination weight rating, or gross vehicle weight or gross combination weight, of 4537 kg (10,001 lb) or more, whichever is greater; or

(2) Is designed or used to transport more than 8 passengers (including the driver) for compensation; or

(3) Is designed or used to transport more than 15 passengers, including the driver, and is not used to transport passengers for compensation; or

(4) Is used in transporting material found by the Secretary of Transportation to be hazardous under 49 U.S.C. 5103 and transported in a quantity requiring placarding under regulations prescribed by the Secretary under 49 CFR, subtitle B, chapter I, subchapter C.

Exempt intracity zone means the geographic area of a municipality or the commercial zone of that municipality described by the FHWA in 49 CFR part 372, subpart B. The descriptions are printed in Appendix F to Subchapter B of this Chapter. The term "exempt intracity zone" does not include any municipality or commercial zone in the State of Hawaii. For purposes of §391.2(d), a driver may be considered to operate a commercial motor vehicle wholly within an exempt intracity zone notwithstanding any common control, management, or arrangement for a continuous carriage or shipment to or from a point without such zone.

Interstate commerce means trade, traffic, or transportation in the United States—

(1) Between a place in a State and a place outside of such State (including a place outside of the United States);

(2) Between two places in a State through another State or a place outside of the United States; or

(3) Between two places in a State as part of trade, traffic, or transportation originating or terminating outside the State or the United States.

Medical examiner means a person who is licensed, certified, and/or registered, in accordance with applicable State laws and regulations, to perform physical examinations. The term includes but is not limited to, doctors of medicine, doctors of osteopathy, physician assistants, advanced practice nurses, and doctors of chiropractic.

PART 391—QUALIFICATIONS OF DRIVERS—
Subpart E—Physical Qualifications and Examinations

Sec. 391.41   Physical qualifications for drivers.

(a) A person shall not drive a commercial motor vehicle unless he/she is physically qualified to do so and, except as provided in Sec. 391.67, has on his/her person the original, or a photographic copy, of a medical examiner's certificate that he/she is physically qualified to drive a commercial motor vehicle.

(b) A person is physically qualified to drive a commercial motor vehicle if that person—

(1) Has no loss of a foot, a leg, a hand, or an arm, or has been granted a skill performance evaluation certificate pursuant to Sec. 391.49;

(2) Has no impairment of:

(i) A hand or finger which interferes with prehension or power grasping; or

(ii) An arm, foot, or leg which interferes with the ability to perform normal tasks associated with operating a commercial motor vehicle; or any other significant limb defect or limitation which interferes with the ability to perform normal tasks associated with operating a commercial motor vehicle; or has been granted a skill performance evaluation certificate pursuant to Sec. 391.49.

(3) Has no established medical history or clinical diagnosis of diabetes mellitus currently requiring insulin for control;

(4) Has no current clinical diagnosis of myocardial infarction, angina pectoris, coronary insufficiency, thrombosis, or any other cardiovascular disease of a variety known to be accompanied by syncope, dyspnea, collapse, or congestive cardiac failure;

(5) Has no established medical history or clinical diagnosis of a respiratory dysfunction likely to interfere with his/her ability to control and drive a commercial motor vehicle safely;

(6) Has no current clinical diagnosis of high blood pressure likely to interfere with his/her ability to operate a commercial motor vehicle safely;

(7) Has no established medical history or clinical diagnosis of rheumatic, arthritic, orthopedic, muscular, neuromuscular, or vascular disease which interferes with his/her ability to control and operate a commercial motor vehicle safely;

(8) Has no established medical history or clinical diagnosis of epilepsy or any other condition which is likely to cause loss of consciousness or any loss of ability to control a commercial motor vehicle;

(9) Has no mental, nervous, organic, or functional disease or psychiatric disorder likely to interfere with his/her ability to drive a commercial motor vehicle safely;

(10) Has distant visual acuity of at least 20/40 (Snellen) in each eye without corrective lenses or visual acuity separately corrected to 20/40 (Snellen) or better with corrective lenses, distant binocular acuity of at least 20/40 (Snellen) in both eyes with or without corrective lenses, field of vision of at least 70 deg. in the horizontal Meridian in each eye, and the ability to recognize the colors of traffic signals and devices showing standard red, green, and amber;

(11) First perceives a forced whispered voice in the better ear at not less than 5 feet with or without the use of a hearing aid or, if tested by use of an audiometric device, does not have an average hearing loss in the better ear greater than 40 decibels at 500 Hz, 1,000 Hz, and 2,000 Hz with or without a hearing aid when the audiometric device is calibrated to American National Standard (formerly ASA Standard) Z24.5—1951.

(12)(i) Does not use a controlled substance identified in 21 CFR 1308.11 Schedule I, an amphetamine, a narcotic, or any other habit-forming drug.

(ii) Exception. A driver may use such a substance or drug, if the substance or drug is prescribed by a licensed medical practitioner who:

(A) Is familiar with the driver's medical history and assigned duties; and

(B) Has advised the driver that the prescribed substance or drug will not adversely affect the driver's ability to safely operate a commercial motor vehicle; and

(13) Has no current clinical diagnosis of alcoholism.

Sec. 391.43   Medical examination; certificate of physical examination.

(a) Except as provided by paragraph (b) of this section, the medical examination shall be performed by a licensed medical examiner as defined in Sec. 390.5 of this subchapter.

(b) A licensed optometrist may perform so much of the medical examination as pertains to visual acuity, field of vision, and the ability to recognize colors as specified in paragraph (10) of Sec. 391.41(b).

(c) Medical examiners shall:

(1) Be knowledgeable of the specific physical and mental demands associated with operating a commercial motor vehicle and the requirements of this **subpart**, including the medical advisory criteria prepared by the FMCSA as guidelines to aid the medical examiner in making the qualification determination; and

(2) Be proficient in the use of and use the medical protocols necessary to adequately perform the medical examination required by this section.

(d) Any driver authorized to operate a commercial motor vehicle within an exempt intracity zone pursuant to Sec. 391.62 of this part shall furnish the examining medical examiner with a copy of the medical findings that led to the issuance of the first certificate of medical examination which allowed the driver to operate a commercial motor vehicle wholly within an exempt intracity zone.

(e) Any driver operating under a limited exemption authorized by Sec. 391.64 shall furnish the medical examiner with a copy of the annual medical findings of the endocrinologist, ophthalmologist or optometrist, as required under that section. If the medical examiner finds the driver qualified under the limited exemption in Sec. 391.64, such fact shall be noted on the Medical Examiner's Certificate.

(f) The medical examination shall be performed, and its results shall be recorded, substantially in accordance with the following instructions and examination form. Existing forms may be used until current printed supplies are depleted or until November 6, 2001, whichever occurs first.

Instructions for Performing and Recording Physical Examinations

The medical examiner must be familiar with 49 CFR 391.41, Physical qualifications for drivers, and should review these instructions before performing the physical examination. Answer each question "yes" or "no" and record numerical readings where indicated on the physical examination form.

The medical examiner must be aware of the rigorous physical, mental, and emotional demands placed on the driver of a commercial motor vehicle. In the interest of public safety, the medical examiner is required to certify that the driver does not have any physical, mental, or organic condition that might affect the driver's ability to operate a commercial motor vehicle safely.

General information. The purpose of this history and physical examination is to detect the presence of physical, mental, or organic conditions of such a character and extent as to affect the driver's ability to operate a commercial motor vehicle safely. The examination should be conducted carefully and should at least include all of the information requested in the following form. History of certain conditions may be cause for rejection. Indicate the need for further testing and/or require evaluation by a specialist. Conditions may be recorded which do not, because of their character or degree, indicate that certification of physical fitness should be denied. However, these conditions should be discussed with the driver and he/she should be advised to take the necessary steps to ensure correction, particularly of those conditions which, if neglected, might affect the driver's ability to drive safely.

General appearance and development. Note marked overweight. Note any postural defect, perceptible limp, tremor, or other conditions that might be caused by alcoholism, thyroid intoxication or other illnesses.

Head-eyes.   When other than the Snellen chart is used, the results of such test must be expressed in values comparable to the standard Snellen test. If the driver wears corrective lenses for driving, these should be worn while driver's visual acuity is being tested. If contact lenses are worn, there should be sufficient evidence of good tolerance of and adaptation to their use. Indicate the driver's need to wear corrective lenses to meet the vision standard on the Medical Examiner's Certificate by checking the box, "Qualified only when wearing corrective lenses." In recording distance vision use 20 feet as normal. Report all vision as a fraction with 20 as the numerator and the smallest type read at 20 feet as the denominator. Monocular drivers are not qualified to operate commercial motor vehicles in interstate commerce.

Ears.   Note evidence of any ear disease, symptoms of aural vertigo, or Meniere's Syndrome. When recording hearing, record distance from patient at which a forced whispered voice can first be heard. For the whispered voice test, the individual should be stationed at least 5 feet from the examiner with the ear being tested turned toward the examiner. The other ear is covered. Using the breath which remains after a normal expiration, the examiner whispers words or random numbers such as 66, 18, 23, etc. The examiner should not use only sibilants (s-sounding test materials). The opposite ear should be tested in the same manner. If the individual fails the whispered voice test, the audiometric test should be administered. For the audiometric test, record decibel loss at 500 Hz, 1,000 Hz, and 2,000 Hz. Average the decibel loss at 500 Hz, 1,000 Hz and 2,000 Hz and record as described on the form. If the individual fails the audiometric test and the whispered voice test has not been administered, the whispered voice test should be performed to determine if the standard applicable to that test can be met.

Throat. Note any irremediable deformities likely to interfere with breathing or swallowing.

Heart. Note murmurs and arrhythmias, and any history of an enlarged heart, congestive heart failure, or cardiovascular disease that is accompanied by syncope, dyspnea, or collapse. Indicate onset date, diagnosis, medication, and any current limitation. An electrocardiogram is required when findings so indicate.

Blood pressure (BP). If a driver has hypertension and/or is being medicated for hypertension, he or she should be recertified more frequently. An individual diagnosed with mild hypertension (initial BP is greater than 160/90 but below 181/105) should be certified for one 3-month period and should be recertified on an annual basis thereafter if his or her BP is reduced. An individual diagnosed with moderate to severe hypertension (initial BP is greater than 180/104) should not be certified until the BP has been reduced to the mild range (below 181/105). At that time, a 3-month certification can be issued. Once the driver has reduced his or her BP to below 161/91, he or she should be recertified every 6 months thereafter. (See Chapter 4 for updated guidelines.)

Lungs. Note abnormal chest wall expansion, respiratory rate, breath sounds including wheezes or alveolar rales, impaired respiratory function, dyspnea, or cyanosis. Abnormal findings on physical exam may require further testing such as pulmonary tests and/or x-ray of chest.

Abdomen and Viscera. Note enlarged liver, enlarged spleen, abnormal masses, bruits, hernia, and significant abdominal wall muscle weakness and tenderness. If the diagnosis suggests that the condition might interfere with the control and safe operation of a commercial motor vehicle, further testing and evaluation is required.

Genital-urinary and rectal examination. A urinalysis is required. Protein, blood or sugar in the urine may be an indication for further testing to rule out any underlying medical problems. Note hernias. A condition causing discomfort should be evaluated to determine the extent to which the condition might interfere with the control and safe operation of a commercial motor vehicle.

Neurological. Note impaired equilibrium, coordination, or speech pattern; paresthesia; asymmetric deep tendon reflexes; sensory or positional abnormalities; abnormal patellar and Babinski's reflexes; ataxia. Abnormal neurological responses may be an indication for further testing to rule out an underlying medical condition. Any neurological condition should be evaluated for the nature and severity of the condition, the degree of limitation present, the likelihood of progressive limitation, and the potential for sudden incapacitation. In instances where the medical examiner has determined that more frequent monitoring of a condition is appropriate, a certificate for a shorter period should be issued.

Spine, musculoskeletal.   Previous surgery, deformities, limitation of motion, and tenderness should be noted. Findings may indicate additional testing and evaluation should be conducted.

Extremities.   Carefully examine upper and lower extremities and note any loss or impairment of leg, foot, toe, arm, hand, or finger. Note any deformities, atrophy, paralysis, partial paralysis, clubbing, edema, or hypotonia. If a hand or finger deformity exists, determine whether prehension and power grasp are sufficient to enable the driver to maintain steering wheel grip and to control other vehicle equipment during routine and emergency driving operations. If a foot or leg deformity exists, determine whether sufficient mobility and strength exist to enable the driver to operate pedals properly. In the case of any loss or impairment to an extremity which may interfere with the driver's ability to operate a commercial motor vehicle safely, the medical examiner should state on the medical certificate "medically unqualified unless accompanied by a Skill Performance Evaluation Certificate." The driver must then apply to the Field Service Center of the FMCSA, for the State in which the driver has legal residence, for a Skill Performance Evaluation Certificate under Sec. 391.49.

Laboratory and Other Testing.   Other test(s) may be indicated based upon the medical history or findings of the physical examination.

Diabetes.   If insulin is necessary to control a diabetic driver's condition, the driver is not qualified to operate a commercial motor vehicle in interstate commerce. If mild diabetes is present and it is controlled by use of an oral hypoglycemic drug and/or diet and exercise, it should not be considered disqualifying. However, the driver must remain under adequate medical supervision.

Upon completion of the examination, the medical examiner must date and sign the form, provide his/her full name, office address and telephone number. The completed medical examination form shall be retained on file at the office of the medical examiner.

(g) If the medical examiner finds that the person he/she examined is physically qualified to drive a commercial motor vehicle in accordance with Sec. 391.41(b), the medical examiner shall complete a certificate in the form prescribed in paragraph (h) of this section and furnish one copy to the person who was examined and one copy to the motor carrier that employs him/her.

(h) The medical examiner's certificate shall be substantially in accordance with the following form. Existing forms may be used until current printed supplies are depleted or until November 6, 2001, whichever occurs first.

Medical Examination Report for Commercial Driver Fitness Determination

Complete form and certificate can be found on pages 30–38.

Pages 4-8 with the exception of 391.41, the medical standards, which are on page 4 of the form, are reproduced here for easier reading

The Driver's Role

Responsibilities, work schedules, physical and emotional demands, and lifestyles among commercial drivers vary by the type of driving that they do. Some of the main types of drivers include the following: turn around or short relay (drivers return to their home base each evening); long relay (drivers drive 8-10 hours and then have an 8-hour off-duty period); straight through haul (cross country drivers); and team drivers (drivers share the driving by alternating their 4-hour driving periods and 4-hour rest periods).

The following factors may be involved in a driver's performance of duties: abrupt schedule changes and rotating work schedules, which may result in irregular sleep patterns and a driver beginning a trip in a fatigued condition; long hours; extended time away from family and friends, which may result in lack of social support; tight pickup and delivery schedules, with irregularity in work, rest, and eating patterns; adverse road, weather and traffic conditions, which may cause delays and lead to hurriedly loading or unloading cargo in order to compensate for the lost time; and environmental conditions such as excessive vibration, noise, and extremes in temperature. Transporting passengers or hazardous materials may add to the demands on the commercial driver.

There may be duties in addition to the driving task for which a driver is responsible and needs to be fit. Some of these responsibilities are: coupling and uncoupling trailer(s) from the tractor, loading and unloading trailer(s) (sometimes a driver may lift a heavy load or unload

Medical Examination Report
FOR COMMERCIAL DRIVER FITNESS DETERMINATION

1. DRIVER'S INFORMATION
Driver completes this section.

| | | | New certification ☐ | Date of Exam |
| Driver's Name (Last, First, Middle) | Social Security No. | Birthdate | Age | Sex | New certification ☐ | Date of Exam |

Driver's Name (Last, First, Middle) | Social Security No. | Birthdate M / D / Y | Age | Sex ☐ M ☐ F | New certification ☐ Recertification ☐ Follow Up ☐ | Date of Exam

| Address | City, State, Zip Code | Work Tel: ( ) Home Tel: ( ) | Driver License No. | License Class ☐ A ☐ C ☐ B ☐ D ☐ Other | State of Issue |

2. HEALTH HISTORY
Driver completes this section, but medical examiner is encouraged to discuss with driver.

Yes No

☐ ☐ Any illness or injury in last 5 years?
☐ ☐ Head/Brain injuries, disorders or illnesses
☐ ☐ Seizures, epilepsy
  ☐ medication
☐ ☐ Eye disorders or impaired vision (except corrective lenses)
☐ ☐ Ear disorders, loss of hearing or balance
☐ ☐ Heart disease or heart attack; other cardiovascular condition
  ☐ medication
☐ ☐ Heart surgery (valve replacement/bypass, angioplasty, pacemaker)
☐ ☐ High blood pressure ☐ medication _____
☐ ☐ Muscular disease
☐ ☐ Shortness of breath

Yes No

☐ ☐ Lung disease, emphysema, asthma, chronic bronchitis
☐ ☐ Kidney disease, dialysis
☐ ☐ Liver disease
☐ ☐ Digestive problems
☐ ☐ Diabetes or elevated blood sugar controlled by:
  ☐ diet
  ☐ pills
  ☐ insulin
☐ ☐ Nervous or psychiatric disorders, e.g., severe depression
  ☐ Medication
☐ ☐ Loss of, or altered consciousness

Yes No

☐ ☐ Fainting, dizziness
☐ ☐ Sleep disorders, pauses in breathing while asleep, daytime sleepiness, loud snoring
☐ ☐ Stroke or paralysis
☐ ☐ Missing or impaired hand, arm, foot, leg, finger, toe
☐ ☐ Spinal injury or disease
☐ ☐ Chronic low back pain
☐ ☐ Regular, frequent alcohol use
☐ ☐ Narcotic or habit forming drug use

For any YES answer, indicate onset date, diagnosis, treating physician's name and address, and any current limitation. List all medications (including over-the-counter medications) used regularly or recently.

_____
_____
_____

I certify that the above information is complete and true. I understand that inaccurate, false or missing information may invalidate the examination and my Medical Examiner's Certificate.

_____   _____
Driver's Signature   Date

Medical Examiners Comments on Health History (The medical examiner must review and discuss with the driver any "yes" answers and potential hazards of medications, including over-the-counter medications, while driving.)

_____
_____
_____
_____

TESTING (Medical Examiner completes Section 3 through 7)

3. VISION

Standard: At least 20/40 acuity (Snellen) in each eye with or without correction. At least 70° peripheral in horizontal meridian measured in each eye. The use of corrective lenses should be noted on the Medical Examiner's Certificate.

INSTRUCTIONS: *When other than the Snellen chart is used, give test results in Snellen-comparable values. In recording distance vision, use 20 feet as normal. Report visual acuity as a ratio with 20 as numerator and the smallest type read at 20 feet as denominator. If the applicant wears corrective lenses, these should be worn while visual acuity is being tested. If the driver habitually wears contact lenses, or intends to do so while driving, sufficient evidence of good tolerance and adaptation to their use must be the obvious. Monocular drivers are not qualified.*

Numerical readings must be provided.

ACUITY	UNCORRECTED	CORRECTED	HORIZONTAL FIELD OF VISION
Right Eye	20/	20/	°
Left Eye	20/	20/	°
Both Eyes	20/	20/	°

Applicant can recognize and distinguish among traffic control signals and devices showing standard red, green, and amber colors? ☐ Yes ☐ No

Applicant meets visual acuity requirement only when wearing:
☐ Corrective Lenses

Monocular Vision: ☐ Yes ☐ No

Complete next line only if vision testing is done by an ophthalmologist or optometrist

Name of Ophthalmologist or Optometrist (print) _____ Tel No. _____ License No./State of Issue _____ Signature _____

Date of Examination _____

4. HEARING

Standard: a) Must first perceive forced whispered voice ≥ 5 ft., with or without hearing aid, or b) average hearing loss in better ear ≤ 40 dB
☐ Check if hearing aid is used for tests.   ☐ Check if hearing aid required to meet standard.

INSTRUCTIONS: *To convert audiometric test results from ISO to ANSI, -14 dB from ISO for 500 Hz, -10 dB for 1,000 Hz, -8.5 dB for 2,000 Hz. To average, add the readings for 3 frequencies tested and divide by 3.*

Numerical readings must be recorded.

	Right Ear	Left Ear
a) Record distance from individual at which forced whispered voice can first be heard.	____ Feet	____ Feet

b) If audiometer is used, record hearing loss in decibels. (acc. to ANSI Z24.5-1951)

	Right Ear			Left Ear		
	500 Hz	1000 Hz	2000 Hz	500 Hz	1000 Hz	2000 Hz
	Average:			Average:		

5. BLOOD PRESSURE / PULSE RATE

Numerical readings must be recorded.

Blood Pressure	Systolic	Diastolic
Driver qualified if ≤ 160/90 on initial exam.		

Pulse Rate	☐ Regular ☐ Irregular

GUIDELINES FOR BLOOD PRESSURE EVALUATION

On initial exam	Within 3 months	Certify
If 161-180 and/or 91-104, Qualify 3 mos. only	If ≤ 160 and/or 90, Qualify for 1 yr. Document Rx & control the 3rd month	Annually if acceptable BP is maintained
If > 180 and/or 104, not qualified until reduced to < 181/105. Then qualify for 3 mos. only.	If ≤ 160 and/or 90, qualify for 6 mos. Document Rx & control the 3rd month	Biannually

Medical examiner should take at least 2 readings to confirm blood pressure.

6. LABORATORY AND OTHER TEST FINDINGS

Numerical readings must be recorded.

Urinalysis is required. Protein, blood or sugar in the urine may be an indication for further testing to rule out any underlying medical problem.

URINE SPECIMEN	SP. GR.	PROTEIN	BLOOD	SUGAR

Other Testing (Describe and record) _____

_____

_____

_____

7. PHYSICAL EXAMINATION

Height: _____ (in.)   Weight: _____ (lbs)

The presence of a certain condition may not necessarily disqualify a driver, particularly if the condition is controlled adequately, is not likely to worsen or is readily amenable to treatment. Even if a condition does not disqualify a driver, the medical examiner may consider deferring the driver temporarily. Also, the driver should be advised to take the necessary steps to correct the condition as soon as possible particularly if the condition, if neglected, could result in more serious illness that might affect driving.

Check YES if there are any abnormalities. Check NO if the body system is normal. Discuss any YES answers in detail in the space below, and indicate whether it would affect the driver's ability to operate a commercial motor vehicle safely. Enter applicable item number before each comment. If organic disease is present, note that it has been compensated for. See *Instructions To The Medical Examiner for guidance.*

BODY SYSTEM	CHECK FOR:	YES*	NO	BODY SYSTEM	CHECK FOR:	YES*	NO
1. General Appearance	Marked overweight, tremor, signs of alcoholism, problem drinking, or drug abuse.			7. Abdomen and Viscera	Enlarged liver, enlarged spleen, masses, bruits, hernia, significant abdominal wall muscle weakness.		
2. Eyes	Pupillary equality, reaction to light, accommodation, ocular motility, ocular muscle imbalance, extraocular movement, nystagmus, exophthalmos, strabismus uncorrected by corrective lenses, retinopathy, cataracts, aphakia, glaucoma, macular degeneration.			8. Vascular system	Abnormal pulse and amplitude, carotid or arterial bruits, varicose veins.		
				9. Genito-urinary system,	Hernias.		
3. Ears	Middle ear disease, occlusion of external canal, perforated eardrums.			10. Extremities - Limb impaired. Driver may be subject to SPE certificate if otherwise qualified.	Loss or impairment of leg, foot, toe, arm, hand, finger. Perceptible limp, deformities, atrophy, weakness, paralysis, clubbing, edema, hypotonia. Insufficient grasp and prehension in upper limb to maintain steering wheel grip. Insufficient mobility and strength in lower limb to operate pedals properly.		
4. Mouth and Throat	Irremediable deformities likely to interfere with breathing or swallowing.						
5. Heart	Murmurs, extra sounds, enlarged heart, pacemaker.			11. Spine, other musculoskeletal	Previous surgery, deformities, limitation of motion, tenderness.		
6. Lungs and chest, not including breast examination.	Abnormal chest wall expansion, abnormal respiratory rate, abnormal breath sounds including wheezes or alveolar rales, impaired respiratory function, dyspnea, cyanosis. Abnormal findings on physical exam may require further testing such as pulmonary tests and/or xray of chest.			12. Neurological	Impaired equilibrium, coordination or speech pattern; paresthesia, asymmetric deep tendon reflexes, sensory or positional abnormalities, abnormal patellar and Babinski's reflexes, ataxia.		

* COMMENTS: _____

_____

_____

Note certification status here. See Instructions to the Medical Examiner for guidance.

☐ Meets standards in 49 CFR 391.41; qualifies for 2 year certificate

☐ Does not meet standards

☐ Meets standards, but periodic evaluation required.

   Due to   driver qualified only for:

    ☐ 3 months   ☐ 1 year

    ☐ 6 months   ☐ Other

☐ Wearing corrective lenses

☐ Wearing hearing aid

☐ Accompanied by a _____ waiver/exemption

☐ Skill Performance Evaluation (SPE) Certificate

☐ Driving within an exempt intracity zone.

☐ Qualified by operation of 49 CFR 391.64

☐ Temporarily disqualified due to (condition or medication): _____

   Return to medical examiner's office for follow up on _____

Medical Examiner's Signature _____

Medical Examiner's Name (print) _____

Address _____

Telephone Number _____

If meets standards, complete a Medical Examiner's Certificate according to 49 CFR 391.43(h). (Driver must carry certificate when operating a commercial vehicle.)

49 CFR 391.41 Physical Qualifications for Drivers

THE DRIVER'S ROLE

Responsibilities, work schedules, physical and emotional demands, and lifestyles among commercial drivers vary by the type of driving that they do. Some of the main types of drivers include the following: turn around or short relay (drivers return to their home base each evening); long relay (drivers drive 8-10 hours and then have an 8-hour off-duty period), straight through haul (cross country drivers); and team drivers (drivers share the driving by alternating their 4-hour driving periods and 4-hour rest periods).

The following factors may be involved in a driver's performance of duties: abrupt schedule changes and rotating work schedules, which may result in irregular sleep patterns and a driver beginning a trip in a fatigued condition; long hours, extended time away from family and friends, which may result in lack of social support; tight pickup and delivery schedules, with irregularity in work, rest, and eating patterns, adverse road, weather and traffic conditions, which may cause delays and lead to hurriedly loading or unloading cargo in order to compensate for the lost time; and environmental conditions such as excessive vibration, noise, and extremes in temperature. Transporting passengers or hazardous materials may add to the demands on the commercial driver.

There may be duties in addition to the driving task for which a driver is responsible and needs to be fit. Some of these responsibilities are: coupling and uncoupling trailer(s) from the tractor, loading and unloading trailer(s) (sometimes a driver may lift a heavy load or unload as much as 50,000 lbs. of freight after sitting for a long period of time without any stretching period); inspecting the operating condition of tractor and trailer(s) before, during, and after delivery of cargo; lifting, installing, and removing heavy tire chains; and, lifting heavy tarpaulins to cover open top trailers. The above tasks demand agility, the ability to bend and stoop, the ability to maintain a crouching position to inspect the underside of the vehicle, frequent entering and exiting of the cab, and the ability to climb ladders on the tractor and/or trailer(s).

In addition, a driver must have the perceptual skills to monitor a sometimes complex driving situation, the judgment skills to make quick decisions, when necessary, and the manipulative skills to control an oversize steering wheel, shift gears using a manual transmission, and maneuver a vehicle in crowded areas.

§ 391.41 PHYSICAL QUALIFICATIONS FOR DRIVERS

(a) A person shall not drive a commercial motor vehicle unless he is physically qualified to do so and, except as provided in §391.67, has on his person the original, or a photographic copy, of a medical examiner's certificate that he is physically qualified to drive a commercial motor vehicle.

(b) A person is physically qualified to drive a motor vehicle if that person:

(1) Has no loss of a foot, a leg, or an arm, or has been granted a Skill Performance Evaluation (SPE) Certificate (formerly Limb Waiver Program) pursuant to §391.49.

(2) Has no impairment of: (i) A hand or finger which interferes with prehension or power grasping; or (ii) An arm, foot, or leg which interferes with the ability to perform normal tasks associated with operating a commercial motor vehicle; or any other significant limb defect or limitation which interferes with the ability to perform normal tasks associated with operating a commercial motor vehicle; or has been granted a SPE Certificate pursuant to §391.49.

(3) Has no established medical history or clinical diagnosis of diabetes mellitus currently requiring insulin for control;

(4) Has no current clinical diagnosis of myocardial infarction, angina pectoris, coronary insufficiency, thrombosis, or any other cardiovascular disease of a variety known to be accompanied by syncope, dyspnea, collapse, or congestive cardiac failure.

(5) Has no established medical history or clinical diagnosis of a respiratory dysfunction likely to interfere with his ability to control and drive a commercial motor vehicle safely.

(6) Has no current clinical diagnosis of high blood pressure likely to interfere with his ability to operate a commercial motor vehicle safely.

(7) Has no established medical history or clinical diagnosis of rheumatic, arthritic, orthopedic, muscular, neuromuscular, or vascular disease which interferes with his ability to control and operate a commercial motor vehicle safely.

(8) Has no established medical history or clinical diagnosis of epilepsy or any other condition which is likely to cause loss of consciousness or any loss of ability to control a commercial motor vehicle;

(9) Has no mental, nervous, organic, or functional disease or psychiatric disorder likely to interfere with his ability to drive a commercial motor vehicle safely;

(10) Has distant visual acuity of at least 20/40 (Snellen) in each eye without corrective lenses or visual acuity separately corrected to 20/40 (Snellen) or better with corrective lenses, distant binocular acuity of at least 20/40 (Snellen) in both eyes with or without corrective lenses, field of vision of at least 70 degrees in the horizontal meridian in each eye, and the ability to recognize the colors of traffic signals and devices showing standard red, green and amber;

(11) First perceives a forced whispered voice in the better ear not less than 5 feet with or without the use of a hearing aid, or, if tested by use of an audiometric device, does not have an average hearing loss in the better ear greater than 40 decibels at 500 Hz, 1,000 Hz and 2,000 Hz with or without a hearing aid when the audiometric device is calibrated to American National Standard (formerly ASA Standard) Z24.5-1951;

(12) (i) Does not use a controlled substance identified in 21 CFR 1308.11 Schedule I, an

amphetamine, a narcotic, or any other habit-forming drug. (ii) Exception: A driver may use such a substance or drug, if the substance or drug is prescribed by a licensed medical practitioner who: (A) Is familiar with the driver's medical history and assigned duties; and (B) Has advised the driver that the prescribed substance or drug will not adversely affect the driver's ability to safely operate a commercial motor vehicle; and

(13) Has no current clinical diagnosis of alcoholism.

General Information

The purpose of this examination is to determine a driver's physical qualification to operate a commercial motor vehicle (CMV) in interstate commerce according to the requirements in 49 CFR 391.41–49. Therefore, the medical examiner must be knowledgeable of these requirements and guidelines developed by the FMCSA to assist the medical examiner in making the qualification determination. The medical examiner should be familiar with the driver's responsibilities and work environment and is referred to the section on the form, The Driver's Role.

In addition to reviewing the Health History section with the driver and conducting the physical examination, the medical examiner should discuss common prescriptions and over-the- counter medications relative to the side effects ad hazards of these medications while driving. Educate driver to read warning labels on all medications. History of certain conditions may be cause for rejection, particularly if required by regulation, or may indicate the need for additional laboratory tests or more stringent examination perhaps by a medical specialist. These decisions are usually made by the medical examiner in light of the driver's job responsibilities, work schedule and potential for the condition to render the driver unsafe.

Medical conditions should be recorded even if they are not cause for denial, and they should be discussed with the driver to encourage appropriate remedial care. This advice is especially needed when a condition, if neglected, could develop into a serious illness that could affect driving.

If the medical examiner determines that the driver is fit to drive and is also able to perform non-driving responsibilities as may be required, the medical examiner signs the medical certificate which the driver must carry with his/her license. The certificate is valid for two years, unless the driver has a medical condition that does not prohibit driving but does require more frequent monitoring. In such situations, the medical certificate should be issued for a shorter length of time. The physical examination should be done carefully and at least as complete as is indicated by the attached form. Contact the FMCSA at (202) 366-1790 for further information (a vision exemption, qualifying drivers under 49 CFR 391.64, etc.).

Interpretation of Medical Standards

Since the issuance of the regulations for physical qualifications of commercial drivers, the Federal Motor Carrier Safety Administration (FMCSA) has published recommendations called Advisory Criteria to help medical examiners in determining whether a driver meets the physical qualifications for commercial driving. These recommendations have been condensed to provide information to medical examiners that (1) is directly relevant to the physical examination form and (2) is not already included in the medical examination form. The specific regulation is printed in italics and its reference by section is highlighted.

Loss of Limb:
§ 391.41(b)(1):

A person is physically qualified to drive a commercial motor vehicle if that person:

Has no loss of a foot, leg, hand or an arm, or has been granted a Skill Performance Evaluation (SPE) Certificate pursuant to Section 391.49.

Limb Impairment:
§ 391.41(b)(2):

A person is physically qualified to drive a commercial motor vehicle if that person:

Has no impairment of: (i) A hand or finger which interferes with prehension or power grasping; or (ii) An arm, foot, or leg which interferes with the ability to perform normal tasks associated with operating a commercial motor vehicle; or (iii) Any other significant limb defect or limitation which interferes with the ability to perform normal tasks associated with operating a commercial motor vehicle; or (iv) Has been granted a Skill Performance Evaluation Certificate pursuant to Section 391.49.

A person who suffers loss of a foot, leg, hand or arm or whose limb impairment in any way interferes with the safe performance of normal tasks associated with operating a commercial motor vehicle is subject to the Skill Performance Evaluation (SPE) Certification Program pursuant to section 391.49, assuming the person is otherwise qualified.

With the advancement of technology, medical aids and equipment modifications have been developed to compensate for certain disabilities. The SPE Certification Program (formerly the Limb Waiver Program) was designed to allow persons with the loss of a foot or limb or with functional impairment to qualify under the Federal Motor Carrier Safety Regulations (FMCSRs) by use of prosthetic devices or equipment modifications which enable them to safely operate a commercial motor vehicle. Since there are no medical aids equivalent to the original body or limb, certain risks are still present, and thus restrictions may be included on individual SPE certificates when a State Director for the FMCSA determines they are necessary to be consistent with safety and public interest.

If the driver is found otherwise medically qualified (391.41(b)(3) through (13)), the medical examiner must check on the medical certificate that the driver is qualified only if accompanied by a SPE certificate. The driver and the employing motor carrier are subject to appropriate penalty if the driver operates a motor vehicle in interstate or foreign commerce without a current SPE certificate for his/her physical disability.

Diabetes
§ 391.41(b)(3)

A person is physically qualified to drive a commercial motor vehicle if that person:

Has no established medical history or clinical diagnosis of diabetes mellitus currently requiring insulin for control.

Diabetes mellitus is a disease which, on occasion, can result in a loss of consciousness or disorientation in time and space. Individuals who require insulin for control have conditions which can get out of control by the use of too much or too little insulin, or food intake not consistent with the insulin dosage. Incapacitation may occur from symptoms of hyperglycemic or hypoglycemic reactions (drowsiness, semiconsciousness, diabetic coma or insulin shock).

The administration of insulin is, within itself, a complicated process requiring insulin, syringe, needle, alcohol sponge and a sterile technique. Factors related to long-haul commercial motor vehicle operations, such as fatigue, lack of sleep, poor diet, emotional conditions, stress, and concomitant illness, compound the diabetic problem. Thus, because of these inherent dangers, the FMCSA has consistently held that a diabetic who uses insulin for control does not meet the minimum physical requirements of the FMCSRs.

Hypoglycemic drugs, taken orally, are sometimes prescribed for diabetic individuals to help stimulate natural body production of insulin. If the condition can be controlled by the use of oral medication and diet, then an individual may be qualified under the present rule.

(See Conference Report on Diabetic Disorders and Commercial Drivers and Insulin-Using Commercial Motor Vehicle Drivers at: *http://www.fmcsa.dot.gov/rulesregs/medreports.htm)*

Cardiovascular Condition
§ 391.41(b)(4)

A person is physically qualified to drive a commercial motor vehicle if that person:

Has no current clinical diagnosis of myocardial infarction, angina pectoris, coronary insufficiency, thrombosis or any other cardiovascular disease of a variety known to be accompanied by syncope, dyspnea, collapse or congestive cardiac failure.

The term "has no current clinical diagnosis of" is specifically designed to encompass: *"a clinical diagnosis of"* (i) a current cardiovascular condition, or (2) a cardiovascular condition which has not fully stabilized regardless of the time limit. The term *"known to be accompanied by"* is defined to include: a clinical diagnosis of a cardiovascular disease (1) which is accompanied by symptoms of syncope, dyspnea, collapse or congestive cardiac failure; and/or (2) which is likely to cause syncope, dyspnea, collapse or congestive cardiac failure.

It is the intent of the FMCSRs to render unqualified a driver who has a current cardiovascular disease which is accompanied by and/or likely to cause symptoms of syncope, dyspnea, collapse, or congestive cardiac failure. However, the subjective decision of whether the nature and severity of an individual's condition will likely cause symptoms of cardiovascular insufficiency is on an individual basis and qualification rests with the medical examiner and the motor carrier. In those cases where there is an occurrence of cardiovascular insufficiency (myocardial infarction, thrombosis, etc.), it is suggested before a driver is certified that he or she have a normal resting and stress electrocardiogram (ECG), no residual complications and no physical limitations, and is taking no medication likely to interfere with safe driving.

Coronary artery bypass surgery and pacemaker implantation are remedial procedures and thus, not necessarily unqualifying. Coumadin is a medical treatment which can improve the health and safety of the driver and should not, by its use, medically disqualify the commercial driver. The emphasis should be on the underlying medical condition(s) which require treatment and the general health of the driver. The FMCSA should be contacted at (202) 366-1790 for additional recommendations regarding the physical qualification of drivers on coumadin.
(See Conference on Cardiac Disorders and Commercial Drivers at: http://www.fmcsa.dot.gov/rulesregs/medreports.htm)

Respiratory Dysfunction
§ 391.41(b)(5)
A person is physically qualified to drive a commercial motor vehicle if that person:
Has no established medical history or clinical diagnosis of a respiratory dysfunction likely to interfere with ability to control and drive a commercial motor vehicle safely.
Since a driver must be alert at all times, any change in his or her mental state is in direct conflict with highway safety. Even the slightest impairment in respiratory function under emergency conditions (when greater oxygen supply is necessary for performance) may be detrimental to safe driving.
There are many conditions that interfere with oxygen exchange and may result in incapacitation, including emphysema, chronic asthma, carcinoma, tuberculosis, chronic bronchitis and sleep apnea. If the medical examiner detects a respiratory dysfunction, that in any way is likely to interfere with the driver's ability to safely control and drive a commercial motor vehicle, the driver must be referred to a specialist for further evaluation and therapy. Anticoagulation therapy for deep vein thrombosis and/or pulmonary thromboembolism is of lower extremity venous optimum dose is achieved, provided lower extremity venous examinations remain normal and the treating physician gives a favorable recommendation.

(See Conference on Pulmonary/Respiratory Disorders and Commercial Drivers at: http://www.fmcsa.dot.gov/rulesregs/medreports.htm)

Hypertension
§ 391.41(b)(6)
A person is physically qualified to drive a commercial motor vehicle if that person:
Has no current clinical diagnosis of high blood pressure likely to interfere with ability to operate a commercial motor vehicle safely.
Hypertension alone is unlikely to cause sudden collapse; however, the likelihood increases when target organ damage, particularly cerebral vascular disease, is present. This regulatory criteria is based on FMCSA's Cardiac Conference recommendations, which used the report of the 1984 Joint National Committee on Detection, Evaluation, and Treatment of High Blood Pressure.
A blood pressure of 161-180 and/or 91-104 diastolic is considered mild hypertension, and the driver is not necessarily unqualified during evaluation and institution of treatment. The driver is given a 3-month period to reduce his or her blood pressure to less than or equal to 160/90; the certifying physician should state on the medical certificate that it is only valid for that 3-month period. If the driver is subsequently found qualified with a blood pressure less than or equal to 160/90, the certifying physician may issue a medical certificate for a 1-year period, but should confirm blood pressure control in the third month of this 1-year period. The individual should be certified annually thereafter. The expiration date must be stated on the medical certificate.
A blood pressure of greater than 180 systolic and/or greater than 104 diastolic is considered moderate to severe. The driver may not be qualified, even temporarily, until his or her blood pressure has been reduced to less than 181/105. The examining physician may temporarily certify the individual once the individual's blood pressure is below 181 and/or 105. For blood pressure greater than 180 and/or 104, documentation of continued control should be made every 6 months. The individual should be certified biannually thereafter. The expiration date must be stated on the medical certificate. Commercial drivers who present for certification with normal blood pressures but are taking medication(s) for hypertension should be certified on the same basis as individuals who present with blood pressures in the mild or moderate to severe range. Annual recertification is recommended if the medical examiner is unable to establish the blood pressure at the time of diagnosis.
An elevated blood pressure finding should be confirmed by at least two subsequent measurements on different days. Inquiry should be made regarding smoking, cardiovascular disease in relatives, and immoderate use of alcohol. An electrocardiogram (ECG) and blood profile, including glucose, cholesterol, HDL cholesterol, creatinine and potassium, should be made. An echocardiogram and chest x-ray are desirable in subjects with moderate or severe hypertension.

Since the presence of target damage increases the risk of sudden collapse, group 3 or 4 hypertensive retinopathy, left ventricular hypertrophy not otherwise explained (echocardiography or ECG by Estes criteria), evidence of severely reduced left ventricular function, or serum creatinine of greater than 2.5 warrants the driver being found unqualified to operate a commercial motor vehicle in interstate commerce.
Treatment includes nonpharmacologic and pharmacologic modalities as well as counseling to reduce other risk factors. Most antihypertensive medications also have side effects, the importance of which must be judged on an individual basis. Individuals must be alerted to the hazards of these medications while driving. Side effects of somnolence or syncope are particularly undesirable in commercial drivers.
A commercial driver who has normal blood pressure 2 or more months after a successful operation for pheochromo- cytoma, primary aldosteronism (unless bilateral adrenalectomy has been performed), renovascular disease, or unilateral renal parenchymal disease, and who shows no evidence of target organ may be qualified. Hypertension that persists despite surgical intervention with no target organ disease should be evaluated and treated following the guidelines set forth above.
(See Conference on Cardiac Disorders and Commercial Drivers at: http://www.fmcsa.dot.gov/rulesregs/medreports.htm)

Rheumatic, Arthritic, Orthopedic, Muscular, Neuromuscular or Vascular Disease
§ 391.41(b)(7)
A person is physically qualified to drive a commercial motor vehicle if that person:
Has no established medical history or clinical diagnosis of rheumatic, arthritic, orthopedic, muscular, neuromuscular or vascular disease which interferes with ability to control and operate a commercial motor vehicle safely.
Certain diseases are known to have acute episodes of transient muscle weakness, poor muscular coordination (ataxia), abnormal sensations (paresthesia), decreased muscular tone (hypotonia), visual disturbances and pain which may be suddenly incapacitating. With each recurring episode, these symptoms may become more pronounced and remain for longer periods of time. Other diseases have more insidious onsets and display symptoms of muscle wasting (atrophy), swelling and paresthesia which may not suddenly incapacitate a person but may restrict his/her movements and eventually interfere with the ability to safely operate a motor vehicle. In many instances these diseases are degenerative in nature or may result in deterioration of the involved area.
Once the individual has been diagnosed as having a rheumatic, arthritic, orthopedic, muscular, neuromuscular or

vascular disease, then he/she has an established history of that disease. The physician, when examining an individual, should consider the following: (1) the nature and severity of that individual's condition (such as sensory loss or loss of strength); (2) the degree of limitation present (such as range of motion); (3) the likelihood of progressive limitation (not always present initially but may manifest itself over time); and (4) the likelihood of sudden incapacitation. If severe functional impairment exists, the driver does not qualify. In cases where more frequent monitoring is required, a certificate for a shorter time period may be issued. (See Conference on Neurological Disorders and Commercial Drivers at: http://www.fmcsa.dot.gov/rulesregs/medreports.htm)

Epilepsy
§ 391.41(b)(8)
A person is physically qualified to drive a commercial motor vehicle if that person:

Has no established medical history or clinical diagnosis of epilepsy or any other condition which is likely to cause loss of consciousness or any loss of ability to control a motor vehicle.

Epilepsy is a chronic functional disease characterized by seizures or episodes that occur without warning, resulting in loss of voluntary control which may lead to loss of consciousness and/or seizures. Therefore, the following drivers cannot be qualified: (1) a driver who has a medical history of epilepsy; (2) a driver who has a current clinical diagnosis of epilepsy; or (3) a driver who is taking antiseizure medication.

If an individual has had a sudden episode of a nonepileptic seizure or loss of consciousness of unknown cause which did not require antiseizure medication, the decision as to whether that person's condition will likely cause loss of consciousness or loss of ability to control a motor vehicle is made on an individual basis by the medical examiner in consultation with the treating physician. Before certification is considered, it is suggested that a 6-month waiting period elapse from the time of the episode. Following the waiting period, it is suggested that the individual have a complete neurological examination. If the results of the examination are negative and antiseizure medication is not required, then the driver may be qualified.

In those individual cases where a driver has a seizure or an episode of loss of consciousness that resulted from a known medical condition (e.g., drug reaction, high temperature, acute infectious disease, dehydration or acute metabolic disturbance), certification should be deferred until the driver has fully recovered from that condition and has no existing residual complications, and not taking antiseizure medication. (See Conference on Neurological Disorders and Commercial Drivers at: http://www.fmcsa.dot.gov/rulesregs/medreports.htm)

Mental Disorders
§ 391.41(b)(9)
A person is physically qualified to drive a commercial motor vehicle if that person:

Has no mental, nervous, organic or functional disease or psychiatric disorder likely to interfere with ability to drive a motor vehicle safely.

Emotional or adjustment problems contribute directly to an individual's level of memory, reasoning, attention and judgment. These problems often underlie physical disorders. A variety of functional disorders can cause drowsiness, dizziness, confusion, weakness or paralysis that may lead to incoordination, inattention, loss of functional control and susceptibility to accidents while driving. Physical fatigue, headache, impaired coordination, recurring physical ailments and chronic "nagging" pain may be present to such a degree that certification for commercial driving is inadvisable. Somatic and psychosomatic complaints should be thoroughly examined when determining an individual's overall fitness to drive. Disorders of a periodically incapacitating nature, even in the early stages of development, may warrant disqualification.

Many bus and truck drivers have documented that "nervous trouble" related to neurotic, personality, emotional or adjustment problems is responsible for a significant fraction of their preventable accidents. The degree to which an individual is able to appreciate, evaluate and adequately respond to environmental strain and emotional stress is critical when assessing an individual's mental alertness and flexibility to cope with the stresses of commercial motor vehicle driving.

When examining the driver, it should be kept in mind that individuals who live under chronic emotional upsets may have deeply ingrained maladaptive or erratic behavior patterns. Excessively antagonistic, instinctive, impulsive, openly aggressive, paranoid or severely depressed behavior greatly interfere with the driver's ability to drive safely. Those individuals who are highly susceptible to frequent states of emotional instability (schizophrenia, affective psychoses, paranoia, anxiety or depressive neurosis) may warrant disqualification. Careful consideration should be given to the side effects and interactions of medications in the overall qualification determination. See Psychiatric Conference Report for specific recommendations on the use of these medications and potential hazards for driving. (See Conference on Psychiatric Disorders and Commercial Drivers at: http://www.fmcsa.dot.gov/rulesregs/medreports.htm)

Vision
§ 391.41(b)(10)
A person is physically qualified to drive a commercial motor vehicle if that person:

Has distant visual acuity of at least 20/40 (Snellen) in each eye with or without corrective lenses or visual acuity separately corrected to 20/40 (Snellen) or better with corrective lenses, distant binocular acuity of at least 20/40 (Snellen) in both eyes with or without corrective lenses, field of vision of at least 70 degrees in the horizontal meridian in each eye, and the ability to recognize the colors of traffic signals and devices showing standard red, green, and amber.

The term "ability to recognize the colors of" is interpreted to mean if a person can recognize and distinguish among traffic control signals and devices showing standard red, green and amber, he or she meets the minimum standard, even though he or she may have some type of color perception deficiency. If certain color perception tests are administered, (such as Ishihara, Pseudoisochromatic, Yarn) and doubtful findings are discovered, a controlled test using signal red, green and amber may be employed to determine the driver's ability to recognize these colors.

Contact lenses are permissible if there is sufficient evidence to indicate that the driver has good tolerance and is well adapted to their use. Use of a contact lens in one eye for distance visual acuity and another lens in the other eye for near vision is not acceptable, nor telescopic lenses acceptable for the driving of commercial motor vehicles.

If an individual meets the criteria by the use of glasses or contact lenses, the following statement shall appear on the Medical Examiner's Certificate: "Qualified only if wearing corrective lenses".

(See Visual Disorders and Commercial Drivers at: http://www.fmcsa.dot.gov/rulesregs/medreports.htm)

Hearing
§ 391.41(b)(11)
A person is physically qualified to drive a commercial motor vehicle if that person:

First perceives a forced whispered voice in the better ear at not less than 5 feet with or without the use of a hearing aid, or, if tested by use of an audiometric device, does not have an average hearing loss in the better ear greater than 40 decibels at 500 Hz, 1,000 Hz, and 2,000 Hz with or without a hearing aid when the audiometric device is calibrated to American National Standard (formerly ASA Standard) Z24.5-1951.

Since the prescribed standard under the FMCSRs is the American Standards Association (ANSI), it may be necessary to convert the audiometric results from the ISO standard to the ANSI standard. Instructions are included on the Medical Examination report form.

If an individual meets the criteria by using a hearing aid, the driver must wear that hearing aid and have it in operation at all times while driving. Also, the driver must be in possession of a spare power source for the hearing aid.

For the whispered voice test, the individual should be stationed at least 5 feet from the examiner with the ear being tested turned toward the examiner. The other ear is covered. Using the breath which remains after a normal expiration, the examiner whispers words or random numbers such as 66, 18, 23, etc. The examiner should not use only sibilants (s-sounding test materials). The opposite ear should be tested in the same manner. If the individual fails the whispered voice test, the audiometric test should be administered.

If an individual meets the criteria by the use of a hearing aid, the following statement must appear on the Medical Examiner's Certificate "Qualified only when wearing a hearing aid".
(See Hearing Disorders and Commercial Motor Vehicle Drivers at: http://www.fmcsa.dot.gov/rulesregs/medreports.htm)

Drug Use
§ 391.41(b)(12)
A person is physically qualified to drive a commercial motor vehicle if that person:
Does not use a controlled substance identified in 21 CFR 1308.11. Schedule I, an amphetamine, a narcotic, or any other habit-forming drug. Exception: A driver may use such a substance or drug, if the substance or drug is prescribed by a licensed medical practitioner who is familiar with the driver's medical history and assigned duties; and has advised the driver that the prescribed substance or drug will not adversely affect the driver's ability to safely operate a commercial motor vehicle.
This exception does not apply to methadone. The intent of the medical certification process is to medically evaluate a driver to ensure that the driver has no medical condition which interferes with the safe performance of driving tasks on a public road. If a driver uses a Schedule I drug or other substance, an amphetamine, a narcotic, or any other habit-forming drug, it may be cause for the driver to be found medically unqualified. Motor carriers are encouraged to obtain a practitioner's written statement about the effects on transportation safety of the use of a particular drug.

A test for controlled substances is not required as part of this biennial certification process. The FMCSA or the driver's employer should be contacted directly for information on controlled substances and alcohol testing under Part 382 of the FMCSRs.

The term "uses" is designed to encompass instances of prohibited drug use determined by a physician through established medical means. This may or may not involve body fluid testing. If body fluid testing takes place, positive test results should be confirmed by a second test of greater

specificity. The term "habit- forming" is intended to include any drug or medication generally recognized as capable of becoming habitual, and which may impair the user's ability to operate a commercial motor vehicle safely.

The driver is medically unqualified for the duration of the prohibited drug(s) use and until a second examination shows the driver is free from the prohibited drug(s) use. Recertification may involve a substance abuse evaluation, the successful completion of a drug rehabilitation program, and a negative drug test result. Additionally, given that the certification period is normally two years, the examiner has the option to certify for a period of less than 2 years if this examiner determines more frequent monitoring is required.
(See Conference on Neurological Disorders and Commercial Drivers and Conference on Psychiatric Disorders and Commercial Drivers at:
http://www.fmcsa.dot.gov/rulesregs/medreports.htm)

Alcoholism
§ 391.41(b)(13)
A person is physically qualified to drive a commercial motor vehicle if that person:
Has no current clinical diagnosis of alcoholism.
The term "current clinical diagnosis of" is specifically designed to encompass a current alcoholic illness or those instances where the individual's physical condition has not fully stabilized, regardless of the time element. If an individual shows signs of having an alcohol-use problem, he or she should be referred to a specialist. After counseling and/or treatment, he or she may be considered for certification.

MEDICAL EXAMINER'S CERTIFICATE

I certify that I have examined _____ in accordance with the Federal Motor Carrier Safety Regulations (49 CFR 391.41-391.49) and with knowledge of the driving duties, I find this person is qualified; and, if applicable, only when:

☐ wearing corrective lenses

☐ wearing hearing aid

☐ accompanied by a _____ waiver/exemption

☐ driving within an exempt intracity zone (49 CFR 391.62)

☐ accompanied by a Skill Performance Evaluation Certificate (SPE)

☐ Qualified by operation of 49 CFR 391.64

The information I have provided regarding this physical examination is true and complete. A complete examination form with any attachment embodies my findings completely and correctly, and is on file in my office.

SIGNATURE OF MEDICAL EXAMINER	TELEPHONE	DATE

MEDICAL EXAMINER'S NAME (PRINT)	☐ MD ☐ DO ☐ Chiropractor
	☐ Physician Assistant ☐ Advanced Practice Nurse

MEDICAL EXAMINER'S LICENSE OR CERTIFICATE NO. / ISSUING STATE

SIGNATURE OF DRIVER	DRIVER'S LICENSE NO.	STATE

ADDRESS OF DRIVER

MEDICAL CERTIFICATE EXPIRATION DATE

as much as 50,000 lbs. of freight after sitting for a long period of time without any stretching period); inspecting the operating condition of tractor and trailer(s) before, during, and after delivery of cargo; lifting, installing, and removing heavy tire chains; and, lifting heavy tarpaulins to cover open top trailers. The above tasks demand agility, the ability to bend and stoop, the ability to maintain a crouching position to inspect the underside of the vehicle, frequent entering and exiting of the cab, and the ability to climb ladders on the tractor and/or trailer(s).

In addition, a driver must have the perceptual skills to monitor a sometimes complex driving situation, the judgment skills to make quick decisions, when necessary, and the manipulative skills to control an oversize steering wheel, shift gears using a manual transmission, and maneuver a vehicle in crowded areas.

Instructions to the Medical Examiner

General Information   The purpose of this examination is to determine a driver's physical qualification to operate a commercial motor vehicle (CMV) in interstate commerce according to the requirements in 49 CFR 391.41-49. Therefore, the medical examiner must be knowledgeable of these requirements and guidelines developed by the FMCSA to assist the medical examiner in making the qualification determination. The medical examiner should be familiar with the driver's responsibilities and work environment and is referred to the section on the form, The Driver's Role.

In addition to reviewing the Health History section with the driver and conducting the physical examination, the medical examiner should discuss common prescriptions and over-the-counter medications relative to the side effects and hazards of these medications while driving. Educate driver to read warning labels on all medications. History of certain conditions may be cause for rejection, particularly if required by regulation, or may indicate the need for additional laboratory tests or more stringent examination perhaps by a medical specialist. These decisions are usually made by the medical examiner in light of the driver's job responsibilities, work schedule and potential for the condition to render the driver unsafe.

Medical conditions should be recorded even if they are not cause for denial, and they should be discussed with the driver to encourage appropriate remedial care. This advice is especially needed when a condition, if neglected, could develop into a serious illness that could affect driving.

If the medical examiner determines that the driver is fit to drive and is also able to perform non-driving responsibilities as may be required, the medical examiner signs the medical certificate which the driver must carry with his/her license. The certificate must be dated. Under current regulations, the certificate is valid for two years, unless the driver has a medical condition that does not prohibit driving but does require more frequent monitoring. In such situations, the medical certificate should be issued for a shorter length of time. The physical examination should be done carefully and at least as complete as is indicated by the attached form.

Contact the FMCSA at (202) 366-1790 for further information (a vision exemption, qualifying drivers under 49 CFR 391.64, etc.).

Interpretation of Medical Standards

Since the issuance of the regulations for physical qualifications of commercial drivers, the Federal Motor Carrier Safety Administration (FMCSA) has published recommendations called Advisory Criteria to help medical examiners in determining whether a driver meets the physical qualifications for commercial driving. These recommendations have been condensed to provide information to medical examiners that (l) is directly relevant to the physical examination and (2) is not already included in the medical examination form. The specific regulation is printed in italics and its reference by section is highlighted.

Federal Motor Carrier Safety Regulations— Advisory Criteria—

Loss of Limb:
§391.41(b)(1)

A person is physically qualified to drive a commercial motor vehicle if that person:

Has no loss of a foot, leg, hand or an arm, or has been granted a Skill Performance Evaluation (SPE) Certificate pursuant to Section 391.49.

Limb Impairment:
§391.41(b)(2)

A person is physically qualified to drive a commercial motor vehicle if that person:

Has no impairment of: (i) A hand or finger which interferes with prehension or power grasping; or (ii) An arm, foot, or leg which interferes with the ability to perform normal tasks associated with operating a commercial motor vehicle; or (iii) Any other significant limb defect or limitation which interferes with the ability to perform normal tasks associated with operating a commercial motor vehicle; or (iv) Has been granted a Skill Performance Evaluation Certificate pursuant to Section 391.49.

A person who suffers loss of a foot, leg, hand or arm or whose limb impairment in any way interferes with the safe performance of normal tasks associated with operating a commercial motor vehicle is subject to the Skill Performance Evaluation (SPE) Certification Program pursuant to section 391.49, assuming the person is otherwise qualified.

With the advancement of technology, medical aids and equipment modifications have been developed to compensate for certain disabilities. The SPE Certification Program (formerly the Limb Waiver Program) was designed to allow persons with the loss of a foot or limb or with functional impairment to qualify under the Federal Motor Carrier Safety Regulations (FMCSRs) by use of prosthetic devices or equipment modifications which enable them to safely operate a commercial motor vehicle. Since there are no medical aids equivalent to the original body or limb, certain risks are still present, and thus restrictions may be included on individual SPE certificates when a State Director for the FMCSA determines they are necessary to be consistent with safety and public interest.

If the driver is found otherwise medically qualified (391.41(b)(3) through (13)), the medical examiner must check on the medical certificate that the driver is qualified only if accompanied by an SPE certificate. The driver and the employing motor carrier are subject to appropriate penalty if the driver operates a motor vehicle in interstate or foreign commerce without a current SPE certificate for his/her physical disability.

Diabetes:
§391.41(b)(3)

A person is physically qualified to drive a commercial motor vehicle if that person:

Has no established medical history or clinical diagnosis of diabetes mellitus currently requiring insulin for control.

Diabetes mellitus is a disease which, on occasion, can result in a loss of consciousness or disorientation in time and space. Individuals who require insulin for control have conditions which can get out of control by the use of too much or too little insulin, or food intake not consistent with the insulin dosage. Incapacitation may occur from symptoms of hyperglycemic or hypoglycemic reactions (drowsiness, semiconsciousness, diabetic coma or insulin shock).

The administration of insulin is, within itself, a complicated process requiring insulin, syringe, needle, alcohol sponge and a sterile technique. Factors related to long-haul commercial motor vehicle operations, such as fatigue, lack of sleep, poor diet, emotional conditions, stress, and concomitant illness, compound the diabetic problem. Thus, because of these inherent dangers, the FMCSA has consistently held that a diabetic who uses insulin for control does not meet the minimum physical requirements of the FMCSRs.

Hypoglycemic drugs, taken orally, are sometimes prescribed for diabetic individuals to help stimulate natural body production of insulin. If the condition can be controlled by the use of oral medication and diet, then an individual may be qualified under the present rule.

(See Conference Report on Diabetic Disorders and Commercial Drivers and Insulin-Using Commercial Motor Vehicle Drivers at: *http:// www.fmcsa.dot.gov/rulesregs/medreports.htm*)

Cardiovascular Condition:
§391.41(b)(4)

A person is physically qualified to drive a commercial motor vehicle if that person:

Has no current clinical diagnosis of myocardial infarction, angina pectoris, coronary insufficiency, thrombosis or any other cardiovascular disease of a variety known to be accompanied by syncope, dyspnea, collapse or congestive cardiac failure.

The term "has no current clinical diagnosis of" is specifically designed to encompass: *"a clinical diagnosis of"* (1) a current cardiovascular condition, or (2) a cardiovascular condition which has not fully stabilized regardless of the time limit. The term *"known to be accompanied by"* is defined to include: *a clinical diagnosis of* a cardiovascular disease (1) which is accompanied by symptoms of syncope, dyspnea, collapse or congestive cardiac failure; and/or (2) which is likely to cause syncope, dyspnea, collapse or congestive cardiac failure.

It is the intent of the FMCSRs to render unqualified a driver who has a current cardiovascular disease which is accompanied by and/or likely to cause symptoms of syncope, dyspnea, collapse, or congestive cardiac failure. However, the subjective decision of whether the nature and severity of an individual's condition will likely cause symptoms of cardiovascular insufficiency is on an individual basis and qualification rests with the medical examiner and the motor carrier. In those cases where there is an occurrence of cardiovascular insufficiency (myocardial infarction, thrombosis, etc.), it is suggested before a driver is certified that he or she have a normal resting and stress electrocardiogram (ECG), no residual complications and no physical limitations, and is taking no medication likely to interfere with safe driving.

Coronary artery bypass surgery and pacemaker implantation are remedial procedures and thus, not unqualifying. Coumadin is a medical treatment which can improve the health and safety of the driver and should not, by its use, medically disqualify the commercial driver. The emphasis should be on the underlying medical condition(s) which require treatment and the general health of the driver. The FMCSA should be contacted at (202) 366-1790 for additional recommendations regarding the physical qualification of drivers on Coumadin.

(See Conference on Cardiac Disorders and Commercial Drivers at: *http://www.fmcsa.dot.gov/rulesregs/medreports.htm*) (See Chapter 4 for updated guidance.)

Respiratory Dysfunction:
§391.41(b)(5)

A person is physically qualified to drive a commercial motor vehicle if that person:

Has no established medical history or clinical diagnosis of a respiratory dysfunction likely to interfere with ability to control and drive a commercial motor vehicle safely.

Since a driver must be alert at all times, any change in his or her mental state is in direct conflict with highway safety. Even the slightest impairment in respiratory function under emergency conditions (when greater oxygen supply is necessary for performance) may be detrimental to safe driving.

There are many conditions that interfere with oxygen exchange and may result in incapacitation, including emphysema, chronic asthma, carcinoma, tuberculosis, chronic bronchitis and sleep apnea. If the medical examiner detects a respiratory dysfunction, that in any way is likely to interfere with the driver's ability to safely control and drive a commercial motor vehicle, the driver must be referred to a specialist for further evaluation and therapy. Anticoagulation therapy for deep vein thrombosis and/or pulmonary thromboembolism is not unqualifying once optimum dose is achieved, provided lower extremity venous examinations remain normal and the treating physician gives a favorable recommendation.

(See Conference on Pulmonary/Respiratory Disorders and Commercial Drivers at: *http://www.fmcsa.dot.gov/rulesregs/medreports.htm*)

Hypertension:
§391.41(b)(6)

A person is physically qualified to drive a commercial motor vehicle if that person:

Has no current clinical diagnosis of high blood pressure likely to interfere with ability to operate a commercial motor vehicle safely.

Hypertension alone is unlikely to cause sudden collapse; however, the likelihood increases when target organ damage, particularly cerebral vascular disease, is present. This regulatory criteria is based on FMCSA's Cardiac Conference recommendations, which used the report of the 1984 Joint National Committee on Detection, Evaluation, and Treatment of High Blood Pressure.

A blood pressure of 161-180 and/or 91-104 diastolic is considered mild hypertension, and the driver is not necessarily unqualified during evaluation and institution of treatment. The driver is given a 3-month period to reduce his or her blood pressure to less than or equal to 160/90; the certifying physician should state on the medical certificate that it is only valid for that 3-month period. If the driver is subsequently found qualified with a blood pressure less than or equal to 160/90, the certifying physician may issue a medical certificate for a 1-year period, but should confirm blood pressure control in the third month of this 1-year period. The individual should be certified annually thereafter. The expiration date must be stated on the medical certificate.

A blood pressure of greater than 180 systolic and/or greater than 104 diastolic is considered moderate to severe. The driver may not be qualified, even temporarily, until his or her blood pressure has been reduced to less than 181/105. The examining physician may temporarily certify the individual once the individual's blood pressure is below 181 and/or 105. For blood pressure greater than 180 and/or 104, documentation of continued control should be made every 6 months. The individual should be certified biannually thereafter. The expiration date must be stated on the medical certificate. Commercial drivers who present for certification with normal blood pressures but are taking medication(s) for hypertension should be certified on the same basis as individuals who present with blood pressures in the mild or moderate to severe range. Annual recertification is recommended if the medical examiner is unable to establish the blood pressure at the time of diagnosis.

An elevated blood pressure finding should be confirmed by at least two subsequent measurements on different days. Inquiry should be made regarding smoking, cardiovascular disease in relatives, and immoderate use of alcohol. An electrocardiogram (ECG) and blood profile, including glucose, cholesterol, HDL cholesterol, creatinine and potassium, should be made. An echocardiogram and chest x-ray are desirable in subjects with moderate or severe hypertension.

Since the presence of target damage increases the risk of sudden collapse, group 3 or 4 hypertensive retinopathy, left ventricular hypertrophy not otherwise explained (echocardiography or ECG by

Estes criteria), evidence of severely reduced left ventricular function, or serum creatinine of greater than 2.5 warrants the driver being found unqualified to operate a commercial motor vehicle in interstate commerce.

Treatment includes nonpharmacologic and pharmacologic modalities as well as counseling to reduce other risk factors. Most antihypertensive medications also have side effects, the importance of which must be judged on an individual basis. Individuals must be alerted to the hazards of these medications while driving. Side effects of somnolence or syncope are particularly undesirable in commercial drivers.

A commercial driver who has normal blood pressure 3 or more months after a successful operation for pheochromocytoma, primary aldosteronism (unless bilateral adrenalectomy has been performed), renovascular disease, or unilateral renal parenchymal disease, and who shows no evidence of target organ (disease) may be qualified. Hypertension that persists despite surgical intervention with no target organ disease should be evaluated and treated following the guidelines set forth above.

(See Conference on Cardiac Disorders and Commercial Drivers at: *http.//www.fmcsa.dot.gov/rulesregs/medreports.htm*) (See Chapter 4 for updated guidance.)

Rheumatic, Arthritic, Orthopedic, Muscular, Neuromuscular or Vascular Disease: §391.41(b)(7)

A person is physically qualified to drive a commercial motor vehicle if that person:

Has no established medical history or clinical diagnosis of rheumatic, arthritic, orthopedic, muscular, neuromuscular or vascular disease which interferes with ability to control and operate a commercial motor vehicle safely.

Certain diseases are known to have acute episodes of transient muscle weakness, poor muscular coordination (ataxia), abnormal sensations (paresthesia), decreased muscular tone (hypotonia), visual disturbances and pain which may be suddenly incapacitating. With each recurring episode, these symptoms may become more pronounced and remain for longer periods of time. Other diseases have more insidious onsets and display symptoms of muscle wasting (atrophy), swelling and paresthesia which may not suddenly incapacitate a person but may restrict his/her movements and eventually interfere with the ability to safely operate a motor vehicle. In many instances these diseases are degenerative in nature or may result in deterioration of the involved area.

Once the individual has been diagnosed as having a rheumatic, arthritic, orthopedic, muscular, neuromuscular or vascular disease, then he/she has an established history of that disease. The physician, when examining an individual, should consider the following: (1) the nature and severity of the individual's condition (such as sensory loss or loss of strength); (2) the degree of limitation present (such as range of motion); (3) the likelihood of progressive limitation (not always present initially but may manifest itself over time); and (4) the likelihood of sudden incapacitation. If severe functional impairment exists, the driver does not qualify. In cases where more frequent monitoring is required, a certificate for a shorter time period may be issued.

(See Conference on Neurological Disorders and Commercial Drivers at: *http://www.fmcsa.dot.gov/rulesregs/medreports.htm*)

Epilepsy:
§391.41(b)(8)

A person is physically qualified to drive a commercial motor vehicle if that person:

Has no established medical history or clinical diagnosis of epilepsy or any other condition which is likely to cause loss of consciousness or any loss of ability to control a motor vehicle.

Epilepsy is a chronic functional disease characterized by seizures or episodes that occur without warning, resulting in loss of voluntary control which may lead to loss of consciousness and/or seizures. Therefore, the following drivers cannot be qualified: (1) a driver who has a medical history of epilepsy; (2) a driver who has a current clinical diagnosis of epilepsy; or (3) a driver who is taking antiseizure medication.

If an individual has had a sudden episode of a nonepileptic seizure or loss of consciousness of unknown cause which did not require antiseizure medication, the decision as to whether that person's condition will likely cause loss of consciousness or loss of ability to control a motor vehicle is made on an individual basis by the medical examiner in consultation with the treating physician. Before certification is considered, it is suggested that a 6-month waiting period elapse from the time of the episode. Following the waiting period, it is suggested that the individual have a complete neurological examination. If the results of the examination are negative and antiseizure medication is not required, then the driver may be qualified.

In those individual cases where a driver has a seizure or an episode of loss of consciousness that resulted from a known medical condition (e.g., drug reaction, high temperature, acute infectious disease, dehydration or acute metabolic disturbance), certification should be deferred until the driver has fully recovered from that condition and has no existing residual complications, and not taking antiseizure medication.

(See Conference on Neurological Disorders and Commercial Drivers at: *http://www.fmcsa.dot.gov/rulesregs/medreports.htm*)

Mental Disorders:
§391.41(b)(9)

A person is physically qualified to drive a commercial motor vehicle if that person:

Has no mental, nervous, organic or functional disease or psychiatric disorder likely to interfere with ability to drive a motor vehicle safely.

Emotional or adjustment problems contribute directly to an individual's level of memory, reasoning, attention and judgment. These problems often underlie physical disorders. A variety of functional disorders can cause drowsiness, dizziness, confusion, weakness or paralysis that may lead to incoordination, inattention, loss of functional control and susceptibility to accidents while driving. Physical fatigue, headache, impaired coordination, recurring physical ailments and chronic "nagging" pain may be present to such a degree that certification for commercial driving is inadvisable. Somatic and psychosomatic complaints should be thoroughly examined when determining an individual's overall fitness to drive. Disorders of a periodically incapacitating nature, even in the early stages of development, may warrant disqualification.

Many bus and truck drivers have documented that "nervous trouble" related to neurotic, personality, emotional or adjustment problems is responsible for a significant fraction of their preventable accidents. The degree to which an individual is able to appreciate, evaluate and adequately respond to environmental strain and emotional stress is critical when assessing an individual's mental alertness and flexibility to cope with the stresses of commercial motor vehicle driving.

When examining the driver, it should be kept in mind that individuals who live under chronic emotional upsets may have deeply ingrained maladaptive or erratic behavior patterns. Excessively antagonistic, instinctive, impulsive, openly aggressive, paranoid or severely depressed behavior greatly interfere with the driver's ability to drive safely. Those individuals who are highly susceptible to frequent states of emotional instability (schizophrenia, affective psychoses, paranoia, anxiety or depressive neuroses) may warrant disqualification. Careful consideration should be given to the side effects and interactions of medications in the overall qualification determination. See Psychiatric Conference Report for specific recommendations on the use of these medications and potential hazards for driving.

(See Conference on Psychiatric Disorders and Commercial Drivers at: *http://www.fmcsa.dot.gov/rulesregs/medreports.htm*)

Vision:
§391.41(b)(10)

A person is physically qualified to drive a commercial motor vehicle if that person:

Has distant visual acuity of at least 20/40 (Snellen) in each eye with or without corrective lenses or visual acuity separately corrected to 20/40 (Snellen) or better with corrective lenses, distant binocular acuity of at least 20/40 (Snellen) in both eyes with or without corrective lenses, field of vision of at least 70 degrees in the horizontal meridian in each eye, and the ability to recognize the colors of traffic signals and devices showing standard red, green, and amber.

The term "ability to recognize the colors of" is interpreted to mean if a person can recognize and distinguish among traffic control signals and devices showing standard red, green and amber, he or she meets the minimum standard, even though he or she may have some type of color perception deficiency. If certain color perception tests are administered (such as Ishihara, Pseudoisochromatic, Yarn) and doubtful findings are discovered, a controlled test using signal red, green and amber may be employed to determine the driver's ability to recognize these colors.

Contact lenses are permissible if there is sufficient evidence to indicate that the driver has good tolerance and is well adapted to their use. Use of a contact lens in one eye for distance visual acuity and another lens in the other eye for near vision is not acceptable, nor (are) telescopic lenses acceptable for the driving of commercial motor vehicles.

If an individual meets the criteria by the use of glasses or contact lenses, the following statement shall appear on the Medical Examiner's Certificate: "Qualified only if wearing corrective lenses."

(See Visual Disorders and Commercial Drivers at: *http://www .fmcsa.dot.gov/rulesregs/medreports.htm*)

Hearing:
§391.41(b)(11)

A person is physically qualified to drive a commercial motor vehicle if that person:

First perceives a forced whispered voice in the better ear at not less than 5 feet with or without the use of a hearing aid, or, if tested by use of an audiometric device, does not have an average hearing loss in the better ear greater than 40 decibels at 500 Hz, 1,000 Hz, and 2,000 Hz with or without a hearing aid when the audiometric device is calibrated to American National Standard (formerly ASA Standard) Z24.5-1951.

Since the prescribed standard under the FMCSRs is the American Standards Association (ANSI), it may be necessary to convert the audiometric results from the ISO standard to the ANSI standard. Instructions are included on the Medical Examination report form.

If an individual meets the criteria by using a hearing aid, the driver must wear that hearing aid and have it in operation at all times while driving. Also, the driver must be in possession of a spare power source for the hearing aid.

For the whispered voice test, the individual should be stationed at least 5 feet from the examiner with the ear being tested turned toward the examiner. The other ear is covered. Using the breath which remains after a normal expiration, the examiner whispers words or random numbers such as 66, 18, 23, etc. The examiner should not use only sibilants (s-sounding test materials). The opposite ear should be tested in the same manner. If the individual fails the whispered voice test, the audiometric test should be administered.

If an individual meets the criteria by the use of a hearing aid, the following statement must appear on the Medical Examiner's Certificate "Qualified only when wearing a hearing aid."

(See Hearing Disorders and Commercial Motor Vehicle Drivers at: *http://www.fmcsa.dot.gov/rulesregs/medreports.htm*)

Drug Use:
§391.41(b)(12)

A person is physically qualified to drive a commercial motor vehicle if that person:

Does not use a controlled substance identified in 21 CFR 1308.11 Schedule I, an amphetamine, a narcotic, or any other habit-forming drug. Exception: A driver may use such a substance or drug, if the substance or drug is prescribed by a licensed medical practitioner who is familiar with the driver's medical history and assigned duties; and has advised the driver that the prescribed substance or drug will not adversely affect the driver's ability to safely operate a commercial motor vehicle.

This exception does not apply to methadone. The intent of the medical certification process is to medically evaluate a driver to ensure that the driver has no medical condition which interferes with the safe performance of driving tasks on a public road. If a driver uses a Schedule I drug or other substance, an amphetamine, a narcotic, or any other habit-forming drug, it may be cause for the driver to be found medically unqualified. Motor carriers are encouraged to obtain a practitioner's written statement about the effects on transportation safety of the use of a particular drug.

A test for controlled substances is not required as part of this biennial certification process. The FMCSA or the driver's employer should be contacted directly for information on controlled substances and alcohol testing under Part 382 of the FMCSRs.

The term "uses" is designed to encompass instances of prohibited drug use determined by a physician through established medical means. This may or may not involve body fluid testing. If body fluid testing takes place, positive test results should be confirmed by a second test of greater specificity. The term "habit-forming" is intended to include any drug or medication generally recognized as capable of becoming habitual, and which may impair the user's ability to operate a commercial motor vehicle safely.

The driver is medically unqualified for the duration of the prohibited drug(s) use and until a second examination shows the driver is free from the prohibited drug(s) use. Recertification may involve a substance abuse evaluation, the successful completion of a drug rehabilitation program, and a negative drug test result. Additionally, given that the certification period is normally two years, the examiner has the option to certify for a period of less than 2 years if this examiner determines more frequent monitoring is required.

(See Conference on Neurological Disorders and Commercial Drivers and Conference on Psychiatric Disorders and Commercial Drivers at: *http://www.fmcsa.dot.gov/rulesregs/medreports.htm*)

Alcoholism:
§391.41(b)(13)

A person is physically qualified to drive a commercial motor vehicle if that person:

Has no current clinical diagnosis of alcoholism.

The term "current clinical diagnosis of" is specifically designed to encompass a current alcoholic illness or those instances where the individual's physical condition has not fully stabilized, regardless of the time element. If an individual shows signs of having an alcohol-use problem, he or she should be referred to a specialist. After counseling and/or treatment, he or she may be considered for certification.

Sec. 391.45   Persons who must be medically examined and certified.

Except as provided in Sec. 391.67, the following persons must be medically examined and certified in accordance with Sec. 391.43 as physically qualified to operate a commercial motor vehicle:

(a) Any person who has not been medically examined and certified as physically qualified to operate a commercial motor vehicle;

(b)(1) Any driver who has not been medically examined and certified as qualified to operate a commercial motor vehicle during the preceding 24 months; or

(2) Any driver authorized to operate a commercial motor vehicle only with an exempt intracity zone pursuant to Sec. 391.62, or only by operation of the exemption in Sec. 391.64, if such driver has not been medically examined and certified as qualified to drive in such zone during the preceding 12 months; and

(c) Any driver whose ability to perform his/her normal duties has been impaired by a physical or mental injury or disease.

Sec. 391.47   Resolution of conflicts of medical evaluation.

(a) Applications. Applications for determination of a driver's medical qualifications under standards in this part will only be accepted if they conform to the requirements of this section.

(b) Content. Applications will be accepted for consideration only if the following conditions are met.

(1) The application must contain the name and address of the driver, motor carrier, and all physicians involved in the proceeding.

(2) The applicant must submit proof that there is a disagreement between the physician for the driver and the physician for the motor carrier concerning the driver's qualifications.

(3) The applicant must submit a copy of an opinion and report including results of all tests of an impartial medical specialist in the field in which the medical conflict arose. The specialist should be one agreed to by the motor carrier and the driver.

(i) In cases where the driver refuses to agree on a specialist and the applicant is the motor carrier, the applicant must submit a statement of his/her agreement to submit the matter to an impartial medical specialist in the field, proof that he/she has requested the driver to submit to the medical specialist, and the response, if any, of the driver to his/her request.

(ii) In cases where the motor carrier refuses to agree on a medical specialist, the driver must submit an opinion and test results of an impartial medical specialist, proof that he/she has requested the motor carrier to agree to submit the matter to the medical specialist and the response, if any, of the motor carrier to his/her request.

(4) The applicant must include a statement explaining in detail why the decision of the medical specialist identified in paragraph (b)(3) of this section, is unacceptable.

(5) The applicant must submit proof that the medical specialist mentioned in paragraph (b)(3) of this section was provided, prior to his/her determination, the medical history of the driver and an agreed-upon statement of the work the driver performs.

(6) The applicant must submit the medical history and statement of work provided to the medical specialist under paragraph (b)(5) of this section.

(7) The applicant must submit all medical records and statements of the physicians who have given opinions on the driver's qualifications.

(8) The applicant must submit a description and a copy of all written and documentary evidence upon which the party making application relies in the form set out in 49 CFR 386.37.

(9) The application must be accompanied by a statement of the driver that he/she intends to drive in interstate commerce not subject to the commercial zone exemption or a statement of the carrier that he/she has used or intends to use the driver for such work.

(10) The applicant must submit three copies of the application and all records.

(c) Information. The Director, Office of Bus and Truck Standards and Operations (MC-PSD) may request further information from the applicant if he/she determines that a decision cannot be made on the evidence submitted. If the applicant fails to submit the information requested, the Director may refuse to issue a determination.

(d)(1) Action. Upon receiving a satisfactory application the Director, Office of Bus and Truck Standards and Operations (MC-PSD) shall notify the parties (the driver, motor carrier, or any other interested party) that the application has been accepted and that a determination will be made. A copy of all evidence received shall be attached to the notice.

(2) Reply. Any party may submit a reply to the notification within 15 days after service. Such reply must be accompanied by all evidence the party wants the Director, Office of Bus and Truck Standards and Operations (MC-PSD) to consider in making his/her determination. Evidence submitted should include all medical records and test results upon which the party relies.

(3) Parties. A party for the purposes of this section includes the motor carrier and the driver, or anyone else submitting an application.

(e) Petitions to review, burden of proof. The driver or motor carrier may petition to review the Director's determination. Such petition must be submitted in accordance with Sec. 386.13(a) of this chapter. The burden of proof in such a proceeding is on the petitioner.

(f) Status of driver. Once an application is submitted to the Director, Office of Bus and Truck Standards and Operations (MC-PSD), the driver shall be deemed disqualified until such time as the Director, Office of Bus and Truck Standards and Operations (MC-PSD) makes a determination, or until the Director, Office of Bus and Truck Standards and Operations (MC-PSD) orders otherwise.

Sec. 391.49   Alternative physical qualification standards for the loss or impairment of limbs.

(a) A person who is not physically qualified to drive under Sec. 391.41(b)(1) or (b)(2) and who is otherwise qualified to drive a commercial motor vehicle, may drive a commercial motor vehicle, if the State Director, FMCSA, has granted a Skill Performance Evaluation (SPE) Certificate to that person.

(b) SPE certificate.—(1) Application. A letter of application for an SPE certificate may be submitted jointly by the person (driver applicant) who seeks an SPE certificate and by the motor carrier that will employ the driver applicant, if the application is accepted.

(2) Application address. The application must be addressed to the applicable field service center, FMCSA, for the State in which the co-applicant motor carrier's principal place of business is located. The address of each, and the States serviced, are listed in Sec. 390.27 of this chapter.

(3) Exception. A letter of application for an SPE certificate may be submitted unilaterally by a driver applicant. The application must be addressed to the field service center, FMCSA, for the State in which the driver has legal residence. The driver applicant must comply with all the requirements of paragraph (c) of this section except those in (c)(1)(i) and (iii). The driver applicant shall respond to the requirements of paragraphs (c)(2)(i) to (v) of this section, if the information is known.

(c) A letter of application for an SPE certificate shall contain:

(1) Identification of the applicant(s):

(i) Name and complete address of the motor carrier coapplicant;

(ii) Name and complete address of the driver applicant;

(iii) The U.S. DOT Motor Carrier Identification Number, if known; and

(iv) A description of the driver applicant's limb impairment for which SPE certificate is requested.

(2) Description of the type of operation the driver will be employed to perform:

(i) State(s) in which the driver will operate for the motor carrier coapplicant (if more than 10 States, designate general geographic area only);

(ii) Average period of time the driver will be driving and/or on duty, per day;

(iii) Type of commodities or cargo to be transported;

(iv) Type of driver operation (i.e., sleeper team, relay, owner operator, etc.); and

(v) Number of years experience operating the type of commercial motor vehicle(s) requested in the letter of application and total years of experience operating all types of commercial motor vehicles.

(3) Description of the commercial motor vehicle(s) the driver applicant intends to drive:

(i) Truck, truck tractor, or bus make, model, and year (if known);

(ii) Drive train;

(A) Transmission type (automatic or manual—if manual, designate number of forward speeds);

(B) Auxiliary transmission (if any) and number of forward speeds; and

(C) Rear axle (designate single speed, 2 speed, or 3 speed).

(iii) Type of brake system;

(iv) Steering, manual or power assisted;

(v) Description of type of trailer(s) (i.e., van, flatbed, cargo tank, drop frame, lowboy, or pole);

(vi) Number of semitrailers or full trailers to be towed at one time;

(vii) For commercial motor vehicles designed to transport passengers, indicate the seating capacity of commercial motor vehicle; and

(viii) Description of any modification(s) made to the commercial motor vehicle for the driver applicant; attach photograph(s) where applicable.

(4) Otherwise qualified:

(i) The coapplicant motor carrier must certify that the driver applicant is otherwise qualified under the regulations of this part;

(ii) In the case of a unilateral application, the driver applicant must certify that he/she is otherwise qualified under the regulations of this part.

(5) Signature of applicant(s):

(i) Driver applicant's signature and date signed;

(ii) Motor carrier official's signature (if application has a coapplicant), title, and date signed. Depending upon the motor carrier's organizational structure (corporation, partnership, or proprietorship), the signer of the application shall be an officer, partner, or the proprietor.

(d) The letter of application for an SPE certificate shall be accompanied by:

(1) A copy of the results of the medical examination performed pursuant to Sec. 391.43;

(2) A copy of the medical certificate completed pursuant to Sec. 391.43(h);

(3) A medical evaluation summary completed by either a board qualified or board certified physiatrist (doctor of physical medicine) or orthopedic surgeon. The coapplicant motor carrier or the driver applicant shall provide the physiatrist or orthopedic surgeon with a description of the job-related tasks the driver applicant will be required to perform;

(i) The medical evaluation summary for a driver applicant disqualified under Sec. 391.41(b)(1) shall include:

(A) An assessment of the functional capabilities of the driver as they relate to the ability of the driver to perform normal tasks associated with operating a commercial motor vehicle; and

(B) A statement by the examiner that the applicant is capable of demonstrating precision prehension (e.g., manipulating knobs and switches) and power grasp prehension (e.g., holding and maneuvering the steering wheel) with each upper limb separately. This requirement does not apply to an individual who was granted a waiver, absent a prosthetic device, prior to the publication of this amendment.

(ii) The medical evaluation summary for a driver applicant disqualified under Sec. 391.41(b)(2) shall include:

(A) An explanation as to how and why the impairment interferes with the ability of the applicant to perform normal tasks associated with operating a commercial motor vehicle;

(B) An assessment and medical opinion of whether the condition will likely remain medically stable over the lifetime of the driver applicant; and

(C) A statement by the examiner that the applicant is capable of demonstrating precision prehension (e.g., manipulating knobs and switches) and power grasp prehension (e.g., holding and maneuvering the steering wheel) with each upper limb separately. This requirement does not apply to an individual who was granted an SPE certificate, absent an orthotic device, prior to the publication of this amendment.

(4) A description of the driver applicant's prosthetic or orthotic device worn, if any;

(5) Road test:

(i) A copy of the driver applicant's road test administered by the motor carrier coapplicant and the certificate issued pursuant to Sec. 391.31(b) through (g); or

(ii) A unilateral applicant shall be responsible for having a road test administered by a motor carrier or a person who is competent to administer the test and evaluate its results.

(6) Application for employment:

(i) A copy of the driver applicant's application for employment completed pursuant to Sec. 391.21; or

(ii) A unilateral applicant shall be responsible for submitting a copy of the last commercial driving position's employment application he/she held. If not previously employed as a commercial driver, so state.

(7) A copy of the driver applicant's SPE certificate of certain physical defects issued by the individual State(s), where applicable; and

(8) A copy of the driver applicant's State Motor Vehicle Driving Record for the past 3 years from each State in which a motor vehicle driver's license or permit has been obtained.

(e) Agreement. A motor carrier that employs a driver with an SPE certificate agrees to:

(1) File promptly (within 30 days of the involved incident) with the Medical Program Specialist, FMCSA service center, such documents and information as may be required about driving activities, accidents, arrests, license suspensions, revocations, or withdrawals, and convictions which involve the driver applicant. This applies whether the driver's SPE certificate is a unilateral one or has a coapplicant motor carrier;

(i) A motor carrier who is a coapplicant must file the required documents with the Medical Program Specialist, FMCSA for the State in which the carrier's principal place of business is located; or

(ii) A motor carrier who employs a driver who has been issued a unilateral SPE certificate must file the required documents with the Medical Program Specialist, FMCSA service center, for the State in which the driver has legal residence.

(2) Evaluate the driver with a road test using the trailer the motor carrier intends the driver to transport or, in lieu of, accept a certificate of a trailer road test from another motor carrier if the trailer type(s) is similar, or accept the trailer road test done during the Skill Performance Evaluation if it is a similar trailer type(s) to that of the prospective motor carrier. Job tasks, as stated in paragraph (e)(3) of this section, are not evaluated in the Skill Performance Evaluation;

(3) Evaluate the driver for those nondriving safety related job tasks associated with whatever type of trailer(s) will be used and any other nondriving safety related or job related tasks unique to the operations of the employing motor carrier; and

(4) Use the driver to operate the type of commercial motor vehicle defined in the SPE certificate only when the driver is in compliance with the conditions and limitations of the SPE certificate.

(f) The driver shall supply each employing motor carrier with a copy of the SPE certificate.

(g) The State Director, FMCSA, may require the driver applicant to demonstrate his or her ability to safely operate the commercial motor vehicle(s) the driver intends to drive to an agent of the State Director,

FMCSA. The SPE certificate form will identify the power unit (bus, truck, truck tractor) for which the SPE certificate has been granted. The SPE certificate forms will also identify the trailer type used in the Skill Performance Evaluation; however, the SPE certificate is not limited to that specific trailer type. A driver may use the SPE certificate with other trailer types if a successful trailer road test is completed in accordance with paragraph (e)(2) of this section. Job tasks, as stated in paragraph (e)(3) of this section, are not evaluated during the Skill Performance Evaluation.

(h) The State Director, FMCSA, may deny the application for SPE certificate or may grant it totally or in part and issue the SPE certificate subject to such terms, conditions, and limitations as deemed consistent with the public interest. The SPE certificate is valid for a period not to exceed 2 years from date of issue, and may be renewed 30 days prior to the expiration date.

(i) The SPE certificate renewal application shall be submitted to the Medical Program Specialist, FMCSA service center, for the State in which the driver has legal residence, if the SPE certificate was issued unilaterally. If the SPE certificate has a coapplicant, then the renewal application is submitted to the Medical Program Specialist, FMCSA field service center, for the State in which the coapplicant motor carrier's principal place of business is located. The SPE certificate renewal application shall contain the following:

(1) Name and complete address of motor carrier currently employing the applicant;

(2) Name and complete address of the driver;

(3) Effective date of the current SPE certificate;

(4) Expiration date of the current SPE certificate;

(5) Total miles driven under the current SPE certificate;

(6) Number of accidents incurred while driving under the current SPE certificate, including date of the accident(s), number of fatalities, number of injuries, and the estimated dollar amount of property damage;

(7) A current medical examination report;

(8) A medical evaluation summary pursuant to paragraph (d)(3) of this section, if an unstable medical condition exists. All handicapped conditions classified under Sec. 391.41(b)(1) are considered unstable. Refer to paragraph (d)(3)(ii) of this section for the condition under Sec. 391.41(b)(2) which may be considered medically stable.

(9) A copy of driver's current State motor vehicle driving record for the period of time the current SPE certificate has been in effect;

(10) Notification of any change in the type of tractor the driver will operate;

(11) Driver's signature and date signed; and

(12) Motor carrier coapplicant's signature and date signed.

(j)(1) Upon granting an SPE certificate, the State Director, FMCSA, will notify the driver applicant and coapplicant motor carrier (if applicable) by letter. The terms, conditions, and limitations of the SPE certificate will be set forth. A motor carrier shall maintain a copy of the SPE certificate in its driver qualification file. A copy of the SPE certificate shall be retained in the motor carrier's file for a period of 3 years after the driver's employment is terminated. The driver applicant shall have the SPE certificate (or a legible copy) in his/her possession whenever on duty.

(2) Upon successful completion of the skill performance evaluation, the State Director, FMCSA, for the State where the driver applicant has legal residence, must notify the driver by letter and enclose an SPE certificate substantially in the following form:

Skill Performance Evaluation Certificate

Name of Issuing Agency: _____

Agency Address: _____

Telephone Number: (   ) _____

Issued Under 49 CFR 391.49, subchapter B of the Federal Motor Carrier Safety Regulations

Driver's Name: _____

Effective Date: _____

SSN: _____

DOB: _____

Expiration Date: _____

Address: _____

_____

_____

Driver Disability: _____

Check One: __New __Renewal

Driver's License: _____
              (State)   (Number)

In accordance with 49 CFR 391.49, subchapter B of the Federal Motor Carrier Safety Regulations (FMCSRs), the driver application for a skill performance evaluation (SPE) certificate is hereby granted authorizing the above-named driver to operate in interstate or foreign commerce under the provisions set forth below. This certificate is granted for the period shown above, not to exceed 2 years, subject to periodic review as may be found necessary. This certificate may be renewed upon submission of a renewal application. Continuation of this certificate is dependent upon strict adherence by the above-named driver to the provisions set forth below and compliance with the FMCSRs. Any failure to comply with provisions herein may be cause for cancellation. CONDITIONS: As a condition of this certificate, reports of all accidents, arrests, suspensions, revocations, withdrawals of driver licenses or permits, and convictions involving the above-named driver shall be reported in writing to the Issuing Agency by the EMPLOYING MOTOR CARRIER within 30 days after occurrence.

LIMITATIONS:

1. Vehicle Type (power unit): _____

2. Vehicle modification(s):_____

_____

3. Prosthetic or Orthotic device(s) (Required to be Worn While Driving): _____

4. Additional Provision(s):_____

NOTICE: To all MOTOR CARRIERS employing a driver with an SPE certificate. This certificate is granted for the operation of the power unit only. It is the responsibility of the employing motor carrier to evaluate the driver with a road test using the trailer type(s) the motor carrier intends the driver to transport, or in lieu of, accept the trailer road test done during the SPE if it is a similar trailer type(s) to that of the prospective motor carrier. Also, it is the responsibility of the employing motor carrier to evaluate the driver for those non-driving safety-related job tasks associated with the type of trailer(s) utilized, as well as, any other non-driving safety-related or job-related tasks unique to the operations of the employing motor carrier.

The SPE of the above named driver was given by a Skill Performance Evaluation Program Specialist. It was successfully completed utilizing the above named power unit and _____ (trailer, if applicable).

The tractor or truck had a _____ transmission.

Please read the NOTICE paragraph above.

Name: _____

Signature: _____

Title: _____

Date: _____

(k) The State Director, FMCSA, may revoke an SPE certificate after the person to whom it was issued is given notice of the proposed revocation and has been allowed a reasonable opportunity to appeal.

(l) Falsifying information in the letter of application, the renewal application, or falsifying information required by this section by either the applicant or motor carrier is prohibited.

Subpart G—Limited Exemptions

Sec. 391.61 Drivers who were regularly employed before January 1, 1971.

The provisions of Sec. 391.21 (relating to applications for employment), Sec. 391.23 (relating to investigations and inquiries), and Sec. 391.33 (relating to road tests) do not apply to a driver who has been a single-employer driver (as defined in Sec. 390.5 of this subchapter) of a motor carrier for a continuous period which began before January 1, 1971, as long as he/she continues to be a single-employer driver of that motor carrier.

Sec. 391.62 Limited exemptions for intra-city zone drivers.

The provisions of Secs. 391.11(b)(1) and 391.41(b)(1) through (b)(11) do not apply to a person who:

(a) Was otherwise qualified to operate and operated a commercial motor vehicle in a municipality or exempt intracity zone thereof throughout the one-year period ending November 18, 1988;

(b) Meets all the other requirements of this section;

(c) Operates wholly within the exempt intracity zone (as defined in 49 CFR 390.5);

(d) Does not operate a vehicle used in the transportation of hazardous materials in a quantity requiring placarding under regulations issued by the Secretary under 49 U.S.C. Chapter 51; and

(e) Has a medical or physical condition which:

(1) Would have prevented such person from operating a commercial motor vehicle under the Federal Motor Carrier Safety Regulations contained in this subchapter;

(2) Existed on July 1, 1988, or at the time of the first required physical examination after that date; and

(3) The examining physician has determined this condition has not substantially worsened since July 1, 1988, or at the time of the first required physical examination after that date.

Sec. 391.63   Multiple-employer drivers.

(a) If a motor carrier employs a person as a multiple-employer driver (as defined in Sec. 390.5 of this subchapter), the motor carrier shall comply with all requirements of this part, except that the motor carrier need not—

(1) Require the person to furnish an application for employment in accordance with Sec. 391.21;

(2) Make the investigations and inquiries specified in Sec. 391.23 with respect to that person;

(3) Perform the annual driving record inquiry required by Sec. 391.25(a);

(4) Perform the annual review of the person's driving record required by Sec. 391.25(b); or

(5) Require the person to furnish a record of violations or a certificate in accordance with Sec. 391.27.

(b) Before a motor carrier permits a multiple-employer driver to drive a commercial motor vehicle, the motor carrier must obtain his/her name, his/her social security number, and the identification number, type and issuing State of his/her commercial motor vehicle operator's license. The motor carrier must maintain this information for three years after employment of the multiple-employer driver ceases.

Sec. 391.64   Grandfathering for certain drivers participating in vision and diabetes waiver study programs.

(a) The provisions of Sec. 391.41(b)(3) do not apply to a driver who was a participant in good standing on March 31, 1996, in a waiver study program concerning the operation of commercial motor vehicles by insulin-controlled diabetic drivers; provided:

(1) The driver is physically examined every year, including an examination by a board-certified/eligible endocrinologist attesting to the fact that the driver is:

(i) Otherwise qualified under Sec. 391.41;

(ii) Free of insulin reactions (an individual is free of insulin reactions if that individual does not have severe hypoglycemia or hypoglycemia unawareness, and has less than one documented, symptomatic hypoglycemic reaction per month);

(iii) Able to and has demonstrated willingness to properly monitor and manage his/her diabetes; and

(iv) Not likely to suffer any diminution in driving ability due to his/her diabetic condition.

(2) The driver agrees to and complies with the following conditions:

(i) A source of rapidly absorbable glucose shall be carried at all times while driving;

(ii) Blood glucose levels shall be self-monitored one hour prior to driving and at least once every four hours while driving or on duty prior to driving using a portable glucose monitoring device equipped with a computerized memory;

(iii) Submit blood glucose logs to the endocrinologist or medical examiner at the annual examination or when otherwise directed by an authorized agent of the FMCSA;

(iv) Provide a copy of the endocrinologist's report to the medical examiner at the time of the annual medical examination; and

(v) Provide a copy of the annual medical certification to the employer for retention in the driver's qualification file and retain a copy of the certification on his/her person while driving for presentation to a duly authorized Federal, State or local enforcement official.

(b) The provisions of Sec. 391.41(b)(10) do not apply to a driver who was a participant in good standing on March 31, 1996, in a waiver study program concerning the operation of commercial motor vehicles by drivers with visual impairment in one eye; provided:

(1) The driver is physically examined every year, including an examination by an ophthalmologist or optometrist attesting to the fact that the driver:

(i) Is otherwise qualified under Sec. 391.41; and

(ii) Continues to measure at least 20/40 (Snellen) in the better eye.

(2) The driver provides a copy of the ophthalmologist or optometrist report to the medical examiner at the time of the annual medical examination.

(3) The driver provides a copy of the annual medical certification to the employer for retention in the driver's qualification file and retains a copy of the certification on his/her person while driving for presentation to a duly authorized federal, state or local enforcement official.

Regulatory Guidance for 49 CFR 391 – Subpart E

Most recently published in Federal Register April 4, 1997 but updated and posted through the FMCSA Website. Guidance for other Subparts can be also be found through *http://www.fmcsa.dot.gov*.

§391.41   Physical Qualifications for Drivers

Question 1: Who is responsible for ensuring that medical certifications meet the requirements?

Guidance: Medical certification determinations are the responsibility of the medical examiner. The motor carrier has the responsibility to ensure that the medical examiner is informed of the minimum medical requirements and the characteristics of the work to be performed. The motor carrier is also responsible for ensuring that only medically qualified drivers are operating CMVs in interstate commerce.

Question 2: Do the physical qualification requirements of the FMCSRs infringe upon a person's religious beliefs if such beliefs prohibit being examined by a licensed doctor of medicine or osteopathy?

Guidance: No. To determine whether a governmental regulation infringes on a person's right to freely practice his religion, the interest served by the regulation must be balanced against the degree to which a person's rights are adversely affected. *Biklen v. Board of Education,* 333 F. Supp. 902 (N.D.N.Y. 1971) aff'd 406 U.S. 951 (1972).

If there is an important objective being promoted by the requirement and the restriction on religious freedom is reasonably adapted to achieving that objective, the requirement should be upheld. *Burgin v. Henderson,* 536 F.2d 501 (2d Cir. 1976).

Based on the tests developed by the courts and the important objective served, the regulation meets Constitutional standards. It does not deny a driver his First Amendment rights.

Question 3: What are the physical qualification requirements for operating a CMV in interstate commerce?

Guidance: The physical qualification regulations for drivers in interstate commerce are found at §391.41. Instructions to medical examiners performing physical examinations of these drivers are found at §391.43. Interpretive guidelines are distributed upon request.

The qualification standards cover 13 areas which directly relate to the driving function. All but four of the standards require a judgment by the medical examiner. A person's qualification to drive is determined by a medical examiner who is knowledgeable about the driver's functions and whether a particular condition would interfere with the driver's ability to operate a CMV safely. In the case of vision, hearing, insulin-using diabetes, and epilepsy, the current standards are absolute, providing no discretion to the medical examiner.

Question 4: Is a driver who is taking prescription methadone qualified to drive a CMV in interstate commerce?

Guidance: Methadone is a habit-forming narcotic which can produce drug dependence and is not an allowable drug for operators of CMVs.

Question 5: May the medical examiner restrict a driver's duties?

Guidance: No. The only conditions a medical examiner may impose upon a driver otherwise qualified involve the use of corrective lenses or hearing aids, securement of a waiver or limitation of driving to exempt intracity zones (see §391.43(g)). A medical examiner who believes a driver has a condition not specified in §391.41 that would affect his ability to operate a CMV safely should refuse to sign the examiner's certificate.

Question 6: If an interstate driver tests positive for alcohol or controlled substances under part 382, must the driver be medically re-examined and obtain a new medical examiner's certificate to drive again?

Guidance: The driver is not required to be medically re-examined or to obtain a new medical examiner's certificate provided the driver is seen by an SAP who evaluates the driver, does not make a clinical diagnosis of alcoholism, and provides the driver with documentation allowing the driver to return to work. However, if the SAP determines that alcoholism exists, the driver is not qualified to drive a CMV in interstate commerce. The ultimate responsibility rests with the motor carrier to ensure the driver is medically qualified and to determine whether a new medical examination should be completed.

Question 7: Are drivers prohibited from using CB radios and earphones?

Guidance: No. CB radios and earphones are not prohibited under the regulations, as long as they do not distract the driver and the driver is capable of complying with §391.41(b)(11).

Question 8: Is the use of Coumadin, an anticoagulant, an automatic disqualification for drivers operating CMVs in interstate commerce?

Guidance: No. Although the FHWA 1987 "Conference on Cardiac Disorders and Commercial Drivers" recommended that drivers who are taking anticoagulants not be allowed to drive, the agency has not adopted a rule to that effect. The medical examiner and treating specialist may, but are not required to, accept the Conference recommendations. Therefore, the use of Coumadin is not an automatic disqualification, but a factor to be considered in determining the driver's physical qualification status.

§391.43   Medical Examination; Certificate of Physical Examination

Question 1: May a motor carrier, for the purposes of §391.41, or a State driver licensing agency, for the purposes of §383.71, accept the results of a medical examination performed by a foreign medical examiner?

Guidance: Yes. Foreign drivers operating in the U.S. with a driver's license recognized as equivalent to the CDL may be medically certified in accordance with the requirements of part 391, subpart E, by a medical examiner in the driver's home country who is licensed, certified, and/or registered to perform physical examinations in that country. However, U.S. drivers operating in interstate commerce within the U.S. must be medically certified in accordance with part 391, subpart E, by a medical examiner licensed, certified, and/or registered to perform physical examinations in the U.S.

Question 2: May a urine sample collected for purposes of performing a subpart H test be used to test for diabetes as part of a driver's FHWA-required physical examination?

Guidance: In general, no. However, the DOT has recognized an exception to this general policy whereby, after 60 milliliters of urine have been set aside for subpart H testing, any remaining portion of the sample may be used for other nondrug testing, but only if such other nondrug testing is required by the FHWA (under part 391, subpart E) such as testing for glucose and protein levels.

Question 3: Is a chest x-ray required under the minimum medical requirements of the FMCSRs?

Guidance: No, but a medical examiner may take an x-ray if appropriate.

Question 4: Does §391.43 of the FMCSRs require that physical examinations of applicants for employment be conducted by medical examiners employed by or designated by the carrier?

Guidance: No.

Question 5: Does a medical certificate displaying a facsimile of a medical examiner's signature meet the "signature of examining health care professional" requirement?

Guidance: Yes.

Question 6: The driver's medical exam is part of the Mexican Licencia Federal. If a roadside inspection reveals that a Mexico-based driver has not had the medical portion of the Licencia Federal re-validated, is the driver considered to be without a valid medical certificate or without a valid license?

Guidance: The Mexican Licencia Federal is issued for a period of 10 years but must be re-validated every 2 years. A condition of re-validation is that the driver must pass a new physical examination. The dates for each re-validation are on the Licencia Federal and must be stamped at the completion of each physical. This constitutes documentation that the driver is medically qualified. Therefore, if the Licencia Federal is not re-validated every 2 years as specified by Mexican law, the driver's license is considered invalid.

Question 7: If a motor carrier sends a potential interstate driver to a medical examiner to have both a pre-employment medical examination and a pre-employment controlled substances test performed, how must the medical examiner conduct the medical examination including the certification the driver meets the physical qualifications of §391.41(b)?

Guidance: The medical examiner must complete the physical examination first without collecting the Part 382 controlled substances urine specimen. If the potential driver meets the requirements of Part 391, Subpart E [especially §391.41(b)] and the medical examiner chooses to certify the potential driver as qualified to operate commercial motor vehicles (CMV) in interstate commerce, the medical examiner may prepare the medical examiner's certificate.

After the medical examiner has completed the medical examiner's certificate and provided a copy to the potential driver and to the motor carrier who will use the potential driver's services, the medical examiner may collect the specimen for the 49 CFR Part 382 pre-employment controlled substances test. The motor carrier is held fully responsible for ensuring the potential driver is not used to operate CMVs until the carrier receives a verified negative controlled substances test result from the medical review officer. A Department of Transportation pre-employment controlled substances test is not a medical examination test.

§391.45   Persons Who Must Be Medically Examined and Certified

Question 1: Is it intended that the words "person" and "driver" be used interchangeably in §391.45?

Guidance: Yes.

Question 2: Do the FMCSRs require applicants, possessing a current medical certificate, to undergo a new physical examination as a condition of employment?

Guidance: No. However, if a motor carrier accepts such a currently valid certificate from a driver subject to part 382, the driver is subject to additional controlled substance testing requirements unless otherwise excepted in subpart H.

Question 3: Must a driver who is returning from an illness or injury undergo a medical examination even if his current medical certificate has not expired?

Guidance: The FMCSRs do not require an examination in this case unless the injury or illness has impaired the driver's ability to perform his/her normal duties. However, the motor carrier may require a driver returning from any illness or injury to take a physical examination. But, in either case, the motor carrier has the obligation to determine if an injury or illness renders the driver medically unqualified.

§391.47   Resolution of Conflicts of Medical Evaluation

Question 1: Does the FHWA issue formal medical decisions as to the physical qualifications of drivers on an individual basis?

Guidance: No, except upon request for resolution of a conflict of medical evaluations.

§391.49   Waiver of Certain Physical Defects

Question 1: Since 49 CFR 391.49 does not mandate a Skill Performance Evaluation, does the term "performance standard" mean that the State must give a driving test or other Skill Performance Evaluation to the driver for every waiver issued or does this term mean that, depending upon the medical condition, the State may give some other type of performance test? For example, in the case of a vision waiver, would a vision examination suffice as a performance standard?

Guidance: Under the Tolerance Guidelines, Appendix C, Paragraph 3(j), each State that creates a waiver program for intrastate drivers is responsible for determining what constitutes "sound medical judgment," as well as determining the performance standard. In the example used above, a vision examination would suffice as a performance standard. It is the responsibility of each State establishing a waiver program to determine what constitutes an appropriate performance standard.

II

Specific Medical Conditions

Natalie P. Hartenbaum, MD, MPH

Most of the regulations that are used to determine whether a commercial driver should be medically qualified can be easily interpreted in several ways. While there are four criteria that are not open to interpretation—vision, hearing, use of insulin, and use of medications to control seizures—the others are intentionally left to the discretion of the medical examiner. When the regulations state that a person should not be certified if a disease "of a variety known to be accompanied by . . ." is present, should the examiner refuse to qualify anyone with a medical diagnosis for which one of the possible outcomes is listed? Or should certification be acceptable unless the risk of sudden incapacitation is almost inevitable?

The intent of these regulations is to balance risk to the public and the driver with the likelihood of a specific event—inability to operate a commercial motor vehicle safely. Many medical conditions can have an impact on driving ability, but usually drivers have sufficient warning to pull their vehicles to the side of the road and prevent an accident.

One component of risk is exposure. While noncommercial drivers often spend less than 3 hours per day behind the wheel, the individuals we are asked to evaluate under 49 CFR 391.41 may be on the road more than 10 hours daily. A neurologic event that has a one in ten chance of occurring during the time a driver of a private vehicle is behind the wheel may have three to four times the likelihood of occurring while a commercial driver is driving. The Canadian Cardiovascular Society uses a 1 percent annual risk of an accident as the defining point at which a commercial driver should not be medically qualified [1].

While the functional status resulting from a chronic disease may not increase the risk for a noncommercial driver, a commercial driver has additional stressors with which to contend (see Part III). Chronic medical problems also may interfere with many of the nondriving tasks of a commercial driver. Musculoskeletal or neurologic impairments may impede the driver's ability to manipulate load-securement devices or maneuver the steering wheel. Most important is the fact that the medical condition may not be present in isolation. A driver with currently stable heart disease and non–insulin-requiring diabetes should be evaluated differently than one with only a single disease process. It is also very important to obtain information from the all treating physicians to assess compliance with treatment and stability of the medical condition(s). If the examiner believes that the driver currently meets the criteria and is safe to operate a commercial vehicle but is uncertain of long-term status, he or she would be well advised to certify the driver for less than 2 years to monitor medical status.

Several references are available to guide the examiner in the decision-making process. The first resource must be the regulations and instructions to examiners, both of which are reproduced in this book (see Chapter 3). The Federal Motor Carrier Safety Administration's advisory criteria provide valuable guidance and are now included on the examination form. While many examiners argue that the conferences sponsored by the Federal Highway Administration (FHWA) are out of date, the recommendations contained in those reports are useful for guidance. Interestingly, many of the recommendations are similar to more recent recommendations from other countries' medical criteria for commercial drivers. These conferences have addressed the commercial driver and such medical conditions as cardiac disorders, pulmonary/respiratory disorders, neurologic disorders, psychiatric disorders, and diabetes. Conference participants included specialists in the particular field, occupational physicians, and representatives from the trucking industry. Other countries and driver licensing agencies also have gathered experts to formulate guidelines.

Apart from studies on fatigue and drug and alcohol use and abuse, there are few studies specifically examining the effects of particular medical conditions on safe driving, and where they do exist, the findings are inconsistent. In this section we have attempted to compile information on specific medical conditions that can be used in evaluating commercial drivers. Much of the information is derived from the FHWA conference reports, and non-U.S. guidelines are included for comparison. Where they exist, conclusions from recent medical literature also are included. Examiners must remember that theirs is the final decision and that good medical judgment, knowledge of disease processes, and an understanding of the driver's roles and responsibilities are all necessary components of the final qualification decision. The information presented is to be used for guidance only. Final decisions, as always, should be based on all available medical information, recent literature, and, most important, good medical judgment.

Reference

1. Brennan FJ, Davies RA, MacDonald RG, et al. Assessment of the cardiac patient for fitness to drive. *Can J Cardiol* 1992;8:406–412.

4

Cardiovascular Disorders

NATALIE P. HARTENBAUM, MD, MPH

Cardiovascular conditions may be one of the most likely medical reasons for sudden incapacitation of a commercial driver. In a 1989 study of 189 fatal-to-driver heavy truck accidents, 10 percent of the accidents were at least in part attributed to medical problems. Of those, 90 percent were cardiac in origin [1]. Studies evaluating the actual increased risk of an accident in drivers with cardiovascular disease are inconsistent. Some [2–3] have found no increased risk, whereas others [4–6] suggest an increased likelihood of a crash in some drivers with cardiovascular disease. Many of these studies focused on the general population and not on commercial drivers. Disease in these individuals may be exacerbated by the long hours, irregular schedules, and physical demands of the job. Many drivers do not perceive driving as stressful, although electrocardiographic (ECG) changes in drivers with heart disease while driving compared with controls have been demonstrated [7–8]. While some drivers with medical conditions that may impair driving skills will limit their driving voluntarily, most do not [9]. In addition to the possibility that cardiovascular disease impairs safe driving in some individuals, one study suggests that commercial drivers have an increased risk of cardiovascular disease compared with the general population [10].

The regulations covering cardiovascular diseases and hypertension are contained in 49 CFR 391.41(b)(4 and 6):

A person is physically qualified to drive a commercial motor vehicle if that person; (4) Has no current clinical diagnosis of myocardial infarction, angina pectoris, coronary insufficiency, thrombosis, or any other cardiovascular disease of a variety known to be accompanied by syncope, dyspnea, collapse, or congestive cardiac failure; (6) Has no current clinical diagnosis of high blood pressure likely to interfere with his/her ability to operate a motor vehicle safely.

Primary care physicians and specialists who are unfamiliar with the Federal Motor Carrier Safety Administration (FMCSA) regulations and other resource information can create conflict and confusion for both patients and examiners. Many examiners have been asked to evaluate a driver whose blood pressure (BP) always runs "just a little high" at 180/105 mm Hg and has been medically qualified by his or her family doctor for the past 20 years. Other examiners have had to explain criteria and conference recommendations to cardiologists who see no reason why a trucker cannot return to work 6 weeks after a myocardial infarction (MI) without further objective testing. There have been studies addressing the knowledge of both cardiologists and family practitioners in local regulations regarding a cardiac patient's ability to drive. In most cases, < 50 percent were aware of existing regulations [11].

Even examiners who are well versed in the issues involved in commercial driver medical certification may interpret the guidelines differently. This is due in part to the vagueness of the advisory criteria and the inconsistency in training and understanding of the issues involved among examiners. The National Transportation Safety Board (NTSB) in 1989 recommended that the Federal Highway Administration (FHWA) develop a clear set of standards for cardiac risk assessment that would be used by medical examiners in evaluating older commercial drivers and all commercial drivers with cardiac conditions. The NTSB also recommended more extensive and frequent evaluations for this group of drivers (NTSB Recommendations H-90-024 and H-90-025) [1].

While the regulations regarding cardiac disease may be open to interpretation, several resources are available for guidance. The Advisory Criteria for the evaluation of commercial drivers should be reviewed first. This can be found on the Medical Reporting Form and will soon be updated to incorporate changes from the new cardiac guidelines. For many years, examiners also relied on the report from the Conference on Cardiac Disorders and Commercial Drivers [12]. Examiners complained that this report, produced with input from cardiologists, industry representatives, and occupational physicians, was older than 13 years. A new set of guidelines was prepared in 2002 and is now available. It can be ordered through the National Technical Information Service (NTIS) at 1-800-533-6847 and will be posted on the FMCSA Internet site. The Cardiovascular Advisory Panel Guidelines for the Medical Examination of Commercial Motor Vehicles Drivers [13] is the focus of this chapter. It has several significant changes, including shortening the waiting period after an MI and directing that, for many conditions, the ejection fraction (EF) should be determined. Implantable defibrillators are also discussed and are believed not to be compatible with commercial driving whether used for primary or secondary prevention. This document is very well written and researched and contains recommendation tables for ease of use. Many of these tables are adapted for use in this chapter. Examiners should review the full report, as the background information is both interesting and useful. This chapter does not cover all of the details or diagnoses but focuses on those that the medical examiner is most likely to encounter. It is explained in the Guidelines that while these are recommendations from the Advisory Panel and are not law, they should be followed. They are intended as standards of practice for medical examiners.

Reports from individual states and other countries can also be reviewed for additional guidance [14–16].

Advisory Criteria

With the new cardiovascular guidelines, the Advisory Criteria will be modified in an upcoming rulemaking for consistency. Much of the content of the current criteria is likely to remain. It explains that the intent of the U.S. Department of Transportation (DOT) is to disqualify those drivers whose medical conditions may predispose them to sudden incapacitation. The criteria suggest that those drivers with a history of coronary insufficiency should be asymptomatic prior to their medical qualification. Recent resting and stress ECGs should be obtained and reviewed. Medications that can affect alertness or cause syncope should be avoided in commercial drivers. The likelihood of a medication exacerbating an underlying arrhythmia also should be assessed.

After coronary artery bypass grafting (CABG), drivers could be medically qualified to drive commercial vehicles provided that (1) their functional capacity is adequate and (2) any medications they may be taking do not cause undesired side effects. The presence of a pacemaker need not automatically be disqualifying. The underlying diagnosis, current cardiac status, and functioning of the pacemaker should be fully evaluated prior to making a decision. Pacemaker function should continue to be monitored to document proper sensing and capture. The examiner is directed to contact 202-366-1970 for additional information on the use of Coumadin. Those recommendations on Coumadin and the commercial motor vehicle driver are included in this chapter but may be updated in light of the new guidelines.

A detailed diagram on determining the qualification of the commercial driver with hypertension is included on the new examination form. This will be updated to be consistent with the new guidelines. The new recommendations for BP are based on the Sixth Report of the Joint National Committee (JNC VI) [17] and can be found in Table 4-1. It is understood that hypertension itself is unlikely to cause collapse; however, there is concern regarding potential end-organ damage and its consequences. For example, the Framingham Study found that in men younger than 65 years, hypertension was the only recognized cardiovascular abnormality associated with sudden death due to atherosclerotic cardiovascular disease. It is also recognized that hypertension is not an all-or-nothing diagnosis and that with increasing arterial pressure, the rates of coronary heart disease and death from all causes increase [18].

Prior to classifying a driver as hypertensive, the BP should be measured on at least three separate occasions with the examinee sitting. If the driver's BP is ≤ 140/90 mm Hg on initial examination and he or she is not taking medication, certification can be for up to 2 years; if the driver is taking medication and BP is ≤ 140/90 mm Hg, he or she should be certified either every 6 months or annually based on BP at the time of diagnosis. If BP is unknown, the advisory criteria had stated that the driver should be examined annually. If the driver has Stage I blood hypertension—systolic BP of 140 to 159 mm Hg and/or diastolic BP of 90 to 99 mm Hg—on initial certification, he or she can be certified to drive for 1 year but should be examined annually, and the BP should be ≤ 140/90 mm Hg at the time of the re-certification examination. If on re-certification examination the BP is < 160/100 mm Hg but > 140/90 mm Hg certification can be extended one time for a 3-month period. Drivers with Stage 2 hypertension—systolic BP of 160 to 179 mm Hg and/or diastolic BP of 100 to 109 mm Hg on initial examination—may be medically certified to drive for one 3-month period, during which treatment should be started. Once the driver has been treated, he or she can be certified for 12 months from the date of the initial examination. Certification should then occur annually, and BP on subsequent examinations should be ≤ 140/90 mm Hg. If the BP at the time of examination is ≥ 180 mm Hg systolic and/or ≥ 110 mm Hg diastolic, the driver should be immediately disqualified until treatment is well tolerated and the BP is ≤ 140/90 mm Hg. Drivers should then be certified for 6 months from the date of the initial examination and every 6 months thereafter. BP should be ≤ 140/90 mm Hg on re-certification examinations.

Hypertensive drivers should also be evaluated and periodically screened for the presence of target-organ damage, including heart failure, stroke, transient ischemic attack, peripheral artery disease, retinopathy, left ventricular hypertrophy, and nephropathy. An examiner

Table 4-1. Recommendations for the commercial driver with hypertension

Diagnosis	Certification	Re-certification
Stage 1 (140–159/90–99 mm Hg)	Yes	Annual BP < 140/90 mm Hg at annual examination; if not but < 160/100 mm Hg, certification extended one time for 3 months
Stage 2 (160–179/100–109 mm Hg)	Yes One-time certification for 3 months Yes, at recheck, if BP ≤ 140/90 mm Hg Certify for 1 year from date of initial examination	Annual BP ≤ 140/90 mm Hg
Stage 3 (≥180/110 mm Hg)	No, immediately disqualifying Yes, at recheck, if BP ≤ 140/90 mm Hg and treatment is well tolerated; certify for 6 months from date of initial examination	Every 6 months BP ≤ 140/90 mm Hg
Secondary hypertension	Based on above stages Yes if: Stage 1 or nonhypertensive ≥ 3 months after surgical correction	Annual BP ≤ 140/90 mm Hg

BP = blood pressure.

Adapted from Blumenthal R, Braunstein J, Connolly H, Epstein A, Gersh BJ, Wittels EH. *Cardiovascular Advisory Panel Guidelines for the Medical Examination of Commercial Motor Vehicles Drivers.* FMCSA-MCP-02-002. Washington: U.S. Department of Transportation, Federal Motor Carrier Safety Administration, October 2002.

could disqualify a driver if target-organ damage impairs the ability to operate the vehicle safely.

The examiner is also advised to review the side effects of any medication used to treat the hypertension. Drivers should be advised about the risk of potentially impairing side effects. It is important to impress on the driver the importance of compliance with medication and treatment beyond allowing him or her to keep the DOT medical card current.

The advisory criteria in effect at the time of publication of this chapter recommends that as part of the initial evaluation of a hypertensive driver, evidence of end-organ damage such as retinopathy or renal insufficiency also should be sought. When grade 3 or 4 hypertensive retinopathy or a creatinine level > 2.5 mg/dL due to hypertension is found, the driver should not be certified. The Advisory Criteria recommend ECG, cholesterol, high-density lipoprotein cholesterol, potassium, and glucose testing. Additionally, drivers with moderate-to-severe hypertension should have a chest x-ray and echocardiogram. This may be modified to reflect current guidelines.

The final issue relating to hypertension in the Advisory Criteria is assessment of an individual after surgery to correct hypertension. This may include surgery for renovascular disease or pheochromocytoma. After surgery, the BP should be controlled, and end-organ damage should be absent. If the driver is still hypertensive after surgery, qualification decisions should be based on the same criteria as discussed previously. This is consistent with new guidelines, but a 3-month wait is advised after surgical correction of secondary hypertension.

Recommendations

The major purpose in evaluating the medical fitness of a commercial driver is to limit potential harm to the general public. The acceptable risk is based on several factors as well as perception. It is difficult to quantify the acceptable risk exactly, but for commercial drivers, exposure, the number of hours on the road, and the severity of the adverse consequence, fatality or injury, must be considered. In most fatal truck accidents, the occupants of passenger vehicles are more likely to be more seriously injured, and, for these reasons, the acceptable risk for commercial drivers should be less than that for drivers of private vehicles [1]. The Canadian Cardiovascular Society suggested that for cardiac disease, the yearly risk for sudden cardiac incapacitation for commercial drivers should be < 1 percent [19].

When performing a commercial driver medical examination, the medical examiner should ask the same cardiac questions as for any other patient. Responses on the history portion of the examination form should be reviewed with the driver. Questions asked should include

Do you have chest pain?

Do you have shortness of breath? With activity? At rest?

Do you have difficulty lying flat at night?

Do you have episodes of dizziness or light-headedness?

Do you have palpitations?

The Advisory Panel suggested that examiners expand the physical examination when coronary heart disease (CHD) disease is present or suspected. Occasionally, the history as offered may not be accurate. Examiners have told me about patients who denied having heart disease on the form, only to reveal on further questioning that they are taking multiple cardiac medications or on examination are found to have prominent chest scars. The Canadian Cardiovascular Society noted that "symptoms may change when some privilege or economic benefit is involved" [19]. While in some cases drivers may be trying to conceal their medical problems, in other cases they may believe that the medications or the surgery corrected their problem and therefore consider the diagnosis no longer current. The new physical examination form requires the driver to sign and certify that the history is accurate.

A thorough physical examination often will yield more information than the history. Some of the physical findings that may suggest cardiac disease include abnormal BP, irregular pulse, distended neck veins, rales, ascites, peripheral edema, and abnormal heart sounds such as gallops or a murmur.

While the Advisory Criteria provide some guidance, detailed and updated guidance is now available in the Cardiovascular Advisory Panel Guidelines [13].

The Canadian Cardiovascular Society recommendations were published in 1991 [19] and updated in 1996 [20]. The Canadian Medical Society prepared a guide, Determining Medical Fitness to Drive in 2000 [14], which is updated regularly on the Internet. The European Society of Cardiology also recently reviewed issues in drivers with heart disease [21]. The remainder of this chapter presents the recommendations of new Advisory Panel guidelines, unless otherwise noted.

Ischemic Heart Disease

Next to hypertension, one of the most common cardiovascular conditions encountered in FMCSA examinations is ischemic heart disease (IHD). It is difficult to determine the exact relationship between IHD and motor vehicle accidents. In one study of 2000 motor vehicle accidents, IHD accounted for 8 percent of accidents caused by driver incapacity [21]. Although 41 percent of deaths from coronary artery disease are sudden, in most cases the driver would have enough warning to pull over to the side of the road to avert an accident [22]. However, one concern would be the occurrence of an arrhythmia in conjunction with the ischemic event, which could be suddenly incapacitating. While most cases of sudden cardiac incapacitation were not associated with serious injury, the consequence of such an event depends on traffic density and the speed of vehicle travel [23].

The evaluation of a driver with coronary artery disease should take into account his or her functional reserve and the risk for arrhythmias. A complete medical history and physical examination must be performed, with special attention given to heart size, rhythm, and rate and the presence or absence of abnormal murmurs, gallops, or pulses. ECGs are no longer routinely recommended and should be obtained only if clinically indicated. There is some suggestion that commercial drivers have an increased number of risk factors for CHD [10, 24]. It was recommended that the examiner obtain information about risk factors by taking a history, from the driver's physician, or through additional testing. Risk factors to be considered are given in Table 4-2. Multiple risk factors alone should not drive the certification decision. Drivers older than 40 years with a Framingham CHD risk for nonfatal MI or CHD death of ≥ 20 percent for 10 years, diabetes mellitus, or peripheral vascular disease (considered to be CHD risk equivalents) are recommended to be evaluated the same as drivers with known CHD. Tables 4-3 and 4-4 are the National Heart, Lung, and Blood Institute Risk Factors tables [25]. It is important to remember that major cardiovascular risk factors, e.g., smoking, elevated BP, elevated serum total cholesterol and low-density lipoprotein cholesterol levels, low serum high-density lipoprotein cholesterol level, diabetes mellitus, and advancing age, are additive. The other major risk factors, i.e., obesity and physical inactivity, are also associated with an increase risk, although their individual and quantitative contributions are not as well defined [26].

Of the nonimaging studies used for predicting future cardiac events, in one study, the most accurate was an inability to achieve 6 metabolic equivalents (METs) on an exercise stress test [27]. Others included a

Table 4-2. Cardiovascular risk factors

Modifiable	Nonmodifiable
Hypertension (systolic BP > 140 mm Hg or diastolic BP > 90 mm Hg)	History of premature heart disease in first-degree relative
Tobacco smoking	Increasing age (> 60 years)
Hypercholesterolemia	Sex (men and postmenopausal women)
Low high-density lipoprotein cholesterol	
Diabetes mellitus	
Overweight or obesity	
Physical inactivity	

BP = blood pressure.

failure to reach 85 percent of maximal predicted heart rate, a 2.0-mm horizontal or down-sloping ST-segment depression in multiple ECG leads, and an inadequate increase in BP during exercise [28]. One study reported that as an independent variable, an increased risk of 1-year mortality was found in those whose EF was < 0.40 or in whom there were > 10 ectopic ventricular depolarizations per hour [29].

The advisory panel did not recommend for or against an exercise tolerance test (ETT) in asymptomatic individuals based on risk factors alone. An examiner may still determine that an ETT is appropriate. The U.S. Preventive Services Task Force does not recommend routine screening by exercise testing for all individuals. In the discussion, however, they acknowledge that for individuals in "certain occupations, such as pilots and heavy equipment operators, where sudden death or incapacitation would endanger the safety of others, considerations other than benefit to the individual patients may favor screening. Although screening cannot reliably identify all persons at risk of an acute event, it may increase the margin of safety for the public" [30]. Each driver should be evaluated on an individual basis, and additional testing should be recommended for those who seem to be at higher risk, and those with the highest risk should be evaluated the same as a driver with CHD.

Table 4-3. Estimate of 10-year risk of myocardial infarction and coronary death for women (Framingham points)

Age	Points
20-34	-7
35-39	-3
40-44	0
45-49	3
50-54	6
55-59	8
60-64	10
65-69	12
70-74	14
75-79	16

Total Cholesterol	Points				
	Age 20-39	Age 40-49	Age 50-59	Age 60-69	Age 70-79
<160	0	0	0	0	0
160-199	4	3	2	1	1
200-239	8	6	4	2	1
240-279	11	8	5	3	2
≥280	13	10	7	4	2

	Points				
	Age 20-39	Age 40-49	Age 50-59	Age 60-69	Age 70-79
Nonsmoker	0	0	0	0	0
Smoker	9	7	4	2	1

HDL (mg/dL)	Points
≥60	-1
50-59	0
40-49	1
<40	2

Systolic BP (mmHg)	If Untreated	If Treated
<120	0	0
120-129	1	3
130-139	2	4
140-159	3	5
≥160	4	6

Point Total	10-Year Risk %
<9	< 1
9	1
10	1
11	1
12	1
13	2
14	2
15	3
16	4
17	5
18	6
19	8
20	11
21	14
22	17
23	22
24	27
≥25	≥ 30

Executive Summary of the Third Report of the National Cholesterol Education Program (NCEP) Expert Panel on the Detection, Evaluation, and Treatment of High Blood Cholesterol in Adults (Adult Treatment Panel III) *http://www.nhlbi.nih.gov/guidelines/cholesterol/atp_iii.htm*. Accessed March 14, 2003.

Table 4-4.   Estimate of 10-year risk of myocardial infarction and coronary death for men (Framingham points)

Age	Points
20-34	-9
35-39	-4
40-44	0
45-49	3
50-54	6
55-59	8
60-64	10
65-69	11
70-74	12
75-79	13

Total Cholesterol	Points				
	Age 20-39	Age 40-49	Age 50-59	Age 60-69	Age 70-79
<160	0	0	0	0	0
160-199	4	3	2	1	0
200-239	7	5	3	1	0
240-279	9	6	4	2	1
≥280	11	8	5	3	1

	Points				
	Age 20-39	Age 40-49	Age 50-59	Age 60-69	Age 70-79
Nonsmoker	0	0	0	0	0
Smoker	8	5	3	1	1

HDL (mg/dL)	Points
≥60	-1
50-59	0
40-49	1
<40	2

Systolic BP (mmHg)	If Untreated	If Treated
<120	0	0
120-129	0	1
130-139	1	2
140-159	1	2
≥160	2	3

Point Total	10-Year Risk %
<0	< 1
0	1
1	1
2	1
3	1
4	1
5	2
6	2
7	3
8	4
9	5
10	6
11	8
12	10
13	12
14	16
15	20
16	25
≥17	≥ 30

Executive Summary of the Third Report of the National Cholesterol Education Program (NCEP) Expert Panel on the Detection, Evaluation, and Treatment of High Blood Cholesterol in Adults (Adult Treatment Panel III) *http:// www.nhlbi.nih.gov/guidelines/cholesterol/atp_iii.htm.* Accessed March 14, 2003.

For those drivers in whom an ETT is appropriate, in those with and without known heart disease, the panel recommended that the driver be able to attain at least 6 METs (through Bruce Stage II or equivalent), have no ischemic changes on exercise ECG, or no ischemic segments on myocardial imaging if performed. They should be able to attain ≥ 85 percent maximum predicted heart rate (unless on beta-blockers), have a rise in systolic BP of ≥ 20 mm Hg without angina, and no significant ST-segment depression or elevation.

Prior to returning to commercial driving after an MI, the driver should be evaluated by a cardiologist, and a 2-month wait is now recommended rather than 3 months. After an MI, the driver should be examined annually and be asymptomatic. One of the new studies recommended is an echocardiogram to assess the EF. This could be performed while still in the hospital, but it should demonstrate an EF of ≥ 40 percent. ETT should be performed 4 to 6 weeks after the MI, and it should be repeated at least every 2 years, more often if indicated. The driver should also not have any side effects from medication, including orthostatic symptoms.

A new definition of MI was published by the Joint European Society/American College of Cardiology Committee in 2000 [31]. The new criteria include those patients with elevated troponin I levels but no elevation of the peak creatinine kinase–MB fraction. More patients who were not considered to have had an MI now meet the criteria. Those who published the new criteria acknowledged that the increased accuracy in diagnosing acute MI may result in consequences for patients, including professional careers. In one study [32], those who were diagnosed by an elevated troponin I level, regardless of ECG changes or creatinine kinase–MB levels, had similar rates of in-hospital events and mortality. They also had a worse, although not statistically significant, 6-month mortality than those diagnosed by the old criteria. This group of patients would not have been identified as having had an acute MI by the old criteria. Even if there is an issue of whether the driver is diagnosed as having had an MI, in this context, they would at least be considered to have unstable angina. If not determined to have had an MI, the certification determination should follow the recommendations for unstable angina.

Angina pectoris is usually caused by narrowing or spasm in one or more coronary arteries. It can either be stable or unstable. If there has not been angina at rest and symptoms have been stable without a change in the pattern of the angina for at least 3 months, the driver can be qualified after examination and approval to drive by a driver's physician, usually a cardiologist. They should have annual qualification examinations and an ETT performed at least every 2 years. In addition, it is recommended that they be asymptomatic both from the disease and from the medications (no light-headedness); no resting systolic BP < 95 mm Hg and no systolic BP decline > 20 mm Hg upon standing.

Percutaneous coronary interventions (PCIs) can be performed in either the acute (MI or unstable angina) or chronic coronary insufficiency setting. If the PCI is performed electively to treat stable angina, the driver could return to work after 1 week with examination and approval of the treating cardiologist. There should be no damage to the vascular site. An ETT is recommended 3 to 6 months after the procedure, with an appropriate result as defined previously. Those drivers who are symptomatic, have an abnormal resting ECG, or are unable to meet the minimum ETT standards should have stress radionuclide or echocardiogram performed. Drivers who have undergone PCIs should have annual medical qualification examinations and a negative ETT at least every 2 years. In addition, it is recommended that they be asymptomatic both from the disease and from the medications (no light-headedness); no resting systolic BP < 95 mm Hg and no systolic BP decline > 20 mm Hg upon standing. If the PCI is performed because of an MI or unstable angina, the recommended waiting period for those conditions should apply.

A waiting period of 3 months is still recommended prior to returning to work as a commercial motor vehicle operator after CABG. This is to allow for sufficient time for sternal wound healing. Examination and approval by a cardiologist should precede return to work, and the driver should undergo annual medical certification examinations. ETTs were not recommended prior to return to work, and there was no specific recommendation as to the frequency of ETTs within 5 years of CABG. When an ETT is performed, the driver should be able to meet the earlier criteria and should not have any ventricular dysrhythmias. The examiner should have a low threshold for requiring radionuclide stress testing or echocardiographic myocardial imaging in these individuals. These are indicated if the driver cannot meet the ETT criteria, has a dysrhythmia, or has an abnormal ECG. A resting echocardiogram is recommended at or prior to the first qualifying examination after the procedure (in-hospital after CABG is acceptable), and the driver's EF should not be < 40 percent. Orthostatic symptoms or other side effects from medications would also be cause for disqualification. Table 4-5 summarizes these recommendations.

Table 4-5. Recommendations for the commercial driver with ischemic heart disease

Diagnosis	Certification	Re-certification
Post-MI	Yes if: ≥2 months post-MI No recurrent anginal symptoms Cleared by a cardiologist Post-MI EF ≥ 40 percent, ETT 4–6 weeks post-MI (completes Stage II of Bruce Protocol—6 METs, 85 percent maximal predicted heart rate, rise in systolic BP ≥20 mm Hg without angina, no significant ST-segment depression, tolerance to medication)	Annual with ETT at least every 2 years If ETT is positive or inconclusive, imaging test recommended Cardiologist evaluation recommended
Angina pectoris	Yes if asymptomatic No if: Change in anginal pattern within 3 months or rest angina, abnormal ETT, ischemic changes on rest ECG, intolerance to medications	Annual, with ETT at least every 2 years If ETT is positive or inconclusive, imaging test recommended Cardiologist evaluation recommended
Post-PCI	Yes if: Not in the setting of MI or unstable angina, at least 1 week after procedure, clearance by a cardiologist and tolerance to medication, no complication at vascular access site, and no ischemic changes on ECG ETT 3–6 months post-PCI	Annual ETT at least every 2 years If ETT is positive or inconclusive, imaging test recommended Cardiologist evaluation recommended

Table 4-5. Recommendations for the commercial driver with ischemic heart disease (*continued*)

Post-CABG	Yes if: ≥ 3 months post-procedure, LVEF ≥ 40 percent, approval by a cardiologist, asymptomatic, and tolerance to medications	Annual After 5 years; annual ETT If ETT is positive or inconclusive, imaging test recommended

BP = blood pressure; CABG = coronary artery bypass grafting; ECG = electrocardiographic; EF = ejection fraction; ETT = exercise tolerance testing; LVEF = left ventricular EF; MET = metabolic equivalent; MI = myocardial infarction; PCI = percutaneous coronary intervention.

Adapted from Blumenthal R, Braunstein J, Connolly H, Epstein A, Gersh BJ, Wittels EH. *Cardiovascular Advisory Panel Guidelines for the Medical Examination of Commercial Motor Vehicle Drivers.* FMCSA-MCP-02-002. Washington: U.S. Department of Transportation, Federal Motor Carrier Safety Administration, FMCSA-MCP-02-002. October 2002.

Hypertension

The hypertension recommendations from the Advisory Panel were reviewed earlier in this chapter. A *Federal Register* announcement will be published to make the applicable changes in the advisory criteria on the examination reporting form.

Valvular Heart Disease

Individuals with valvular heart disease will have degrees of disability ranging from none to severe impairment. The Advisory Panel drew many of their recommendations from the American College of Cardiology (ACC)/American Heart Association (AHA) Guidelines for the Management of Patients with Valvular Heart Disease [33]. Evaluation should be by a cardiologist and with initial evaluation including a history, physical examination, and ECG, and in many patients a chest x-ray. Depending on the specific diagnosis, ECG or ETT may be indicated.

Mitral Stenosis. In addition to the standard initial evaluation, 2-dimensional Doppler echocardiography should be performed. Stress testing may be indicated to assess effort tolerance and the effect of the stenosis on functional capacity. The normal mitral valve area is 4 to 6 cm^2, with severe mitral stenosis defined as a valve area of ≤ 1.0 cm^2, a resting mean pressure gradient of ≥ 10 mm Hg, or a pressure half-time of ≥ 220 msec. Symptoms, the presence of atrial fibrillation, or systolic embolization should also be considered in addition to valve area. Drivers with either mild or moderate mitral stenosis can be certified annually if they are asymptomatic. They should be evaluated annually by a cardiologist, and a 2-dimensional Doppler echocardiography would usually be appropriate. Drivers should be disqualified if their symptoms place them in New York Heart Association Class II or higher (Table 4-6), they have paroxysmal or established atrial fibrillation, or they have a history of systolic embolization. If the pulmonary artery pressure is ≥ 50 percent of systemic pressure or the driver is unable to exercise for > 6 METs on Bruce protocol ETT, they also should not be certified. If a percutaneous balloon valvuloplasty is performed, the driver could be certified after at least a 4-week wait or after at least a 3-month wait for a surgical commissurotomy provided there are no thromboembolic complications after surgery and pulmonary artery pressure is not ≥ 50 percent of systemic BP. In either circumstance, the driver should be re-certified annually with an annual evaluation by a cardiologist.

Mitral Regurgitation.   The standard initial evaluation is a chest x-ray and a two-dimensional Doppler echocardiogram. Stress testing should be obtained if needed to assess effort tolerance and symptomatic status if unclear. In some cases, transesophageal echocardiography may be appropriate. Drivers with severe mitral regurgitation who are symptomatic or have reduced effort tolerance (≤ 6 METs or ≤ 6 minutes

Table 4-6.	New York Heart Association functional capacity
Class I	Cardiac disease but no limitations of physical activity.
Class II	Cardiac disease resulting in slight limitation of physical activity. Comfortable at rest. Ordinary physical activity results in fatigue, palpitations, dyspnea, or anginal pain.
Class III	Cardiac disease resulting in marked limitation of physical activity. Comfortable at rest. Less than ordinary activity causes fatigue, palpitation, dyspnea, or anginal pain.
Class IV	Cardiac disease resulting in inability to carry on any physical activity without discomfort. Symptoms of heart failure or the anginal syndrome may be present even at rest. If any physical activity is undertaken, discomfort increases.

American Heart Association. *http://www.americanheart.org.* Accessed March 14, 2003.

on a Bruce protocol), ruptured chordae or flail leaflet, atrial fibrillation, or thromboembolism should be disqualified. Other recommendations for disqualification include left ventricular dysfunction (EF < 60 percent or left ventricular end systolic dimension > 45 mm or left ventricular end diastolic dimension ≥ 70 mm) or pulmonary hypertension (pulmonary artery pressure > 50 percent systemic arterial pressure). Those with severe mitral regurgitation who are asymptomatic and do not meet the previously mentioned disqualifying criteria can be medically qualified but should be re-certified annually with an echocardiogram every 6 to 12 months and stress testing to assess effort tolerance. Those with mild or moderate mitral regurgitation can be qualified if they are asymptomatic, have normal left ventricular size and function, and have normal pulmonary artery pressure. They should be re-certified annually. Annual echocardiography is not required with mild regurgitation but is indicated annually for those with moderate disease.

If the individual has undergone surgical repair of the mitral valve, there should be at least a 3-month waiting period after the procedure. For follow-up certifications, drivers should be asymptomatic.

Aortic Stenosis. Patients with aortic stenosis tend to do well during a latent period, during which they may be asymptomatic. Once symptoms of angina, syncope, or congestive heart failure develop, prognosis is poor, with survival of < 3 years. Sudden death has also been seen in patients with aortic stenosis who were asymptomatic but with a positive stress test and a valve area of ≤ 0.6 cm^2 [34]. The initial evaluation should include the history and physical examination, ECG, and 2-dimensional Doppler echocardiography to assess gradient, valve area, and severity of left ventricular hypertrophy. Cardiac catheterization and coronary angiography may be needed, and ETT is occasionally required to assess symptoms, effort tolerance, and prognosis. Table 4-7 contains the recommendations for the commercial driver with aortic stenosis.

Aortic Regurgitation. In addition to the standard evaluation, chest x-ray and 2-dimensional echocardiography should be obtained. ETT may be useful for those who are sedentary or if symptoms are equivocal. Drivers with severe aortic regurgitation should be disqualified if they are symptomatic or unable to obtain > 6 METs on ETT, have a reduced EF ≤ 50 percent, or if they have an end systolic dimension > 55 mm or end diastolic dimension 70 mm with normal EF or if they are in atrial fibrillation. A second examination by a cardiologist is recommended 2 to 3 months after the initial evaluation to determine whether there has been progression of the condition. Drivers who are asymptomatic with

Table 4-7. Recommendations for the commercial driver with aortic stenosis

Diagnosis	Certification	Re-certification
Mild aortic stenosis (AVA ≥1.5 cm²)	Yes, if asymptomatic	Annual Echocardiogram every 5 years
Moderate aortic stenosis (AVA ≥ 1.0-1.5 cm²)	Yes if asymptomatic	Annual Echocardiogram every 1–2 years
	Yes if ≥ 3 months after surgery	Annual
	No if: Angina; heart failure; syncope; atrial fibrillation; LV dysfunction with EF < 50 percent; thromboembolism	
Severe aortic stenosis (AVA < 1.0 cm²)	No, irrespective of symptoms or LV function	
	Yes, if ≥ 3 months after surgery	Annual

AVA = aortic valve area; EF = ejection fraction; LV = left ventricular.

Adapted from Blumenthal R, Braunstein J, Connolly H, Epstein A, Gersh BJ, Wittels EH. *Cardiovascular Advisory Panel Guidelines for the Medical Examination of Commercial Motor Vehicle Drivers.* FMCSA-MCP-02-002. Washington: U.S. Department of Transportation, Federal Motor Carrier Safety Administration, October 2002.

mild or moderate aortic regurgitation should be re-certified annually with an echocardiogram every 2 to 3 years. For severe disease, refer to Table 4-8. After valve repair there should be a 3-month waiting period, clearance by a cardiologist, and no thromboembolic complications.

Prosthetic Valve Repair. After valve repair with a mechanical prosthetic valve, commercial drivers can return to work after at least a 3-month wait and clearance by a cardiologist provided they are

Table 4-8. Recommendations for the commercial driver with aortic regurgitation

Diagnosis	Certification	Re-certification
Mild aortic regurgitation	Yes if asymptomatic	Annual Echocardiogram every 2–3 years
Moderate aortic regurgitation	Yes if: Normal LV function No or mild LV enlargement	Annual Echocardiogram every 2–3 years
Severe aortic regurgitation	Yes if: Asymptomatic Normal LV function (EF ≥ 50 percent) LV dilatation LVEDD <60mm LVESD <50 mm	Every 6 months Echocardiogram every 6–12 months
	If LVEDD ≥ 60 mm or LVESD ≥ 50 mm: No if: Symptoms Unable to complete Stage II of Bruce protocol Reduced EF < 50 percent LV dilatation LVEDD > 70mm or LVESD > 55 mm Yes if: Valve surgery and ≥ 3 months since surgery Asymptomatic and cleared by cardiologist	Every 4–6 months Echocardiogram every 4–6 months if no surgery performed

Annual |

EF = ejection fraction; LV = left ventricular; LVEDD = LV end diastolic dimension; LVESD = LV end systolic dimension.

Adapted from Blumenthal R, Braunstein J, Connolly H, Epstein A, Gersh BJ, Wittels EH. *Cardiovascular Advisory Panel Guidelines for the Medical Examination of Commercial Motor Vehicle Drivers.* FMCSA-MCP-02-002. Washington: U.S. Department of Transportation, Federal Motor Carrier Safety Administration, FMCSA-MCP-02-002. October 2002.

asymptomatic. They should not be qualified if they have left ventricular dysfunction (EF < 40 percent), thromboembolic complications postprocedure, or pulmonary hypertension or if they are unable to maintain adequate anticoagulation. The international normalized ratio (INR) should be monitored monthly. If a biologic prosthetic valve is used, the same criteria should be used except that anticoagulation is not necessary if there is no history of emboli or a hypercoagulable state. Those drivers who have atrial fibrillation after valve repair can be certified after the appropriate waiting period and if they are adequately anticoagulated for at least 1 month and monitored monthly by INR. The rate should be controlled and they should be cleared by a cardiologist.

Myocardial Disease

Drivers with echocardiographically diagnosed hypertrophic cardiomyopathy should not be qualified. Those with borderline hypertrophic cardiomyopathy, hypertensive hypertrophic cardiomyopathy, or other similar diagnoses could be qualified but should be reevaluated after 1 year. Owing to a poor prognosis, drivers with restrictive cardiomyopathy should be disqualified.

Drivers with congestive cardiac failure or idiopathic dilated cardiomyopathy and an EF of < 40 percent should be disqualified. If a subsequent evaluation demonstrates an improved EF ≥ 40 percent, the driver can be re-certified if asymptomatic. Evaluation should include 2-dimensional Doppler echocardiography to assess EF, left ventricular size, and/or valvular heart disease. Radionuclide ventriculography or ETT may be indicated in some patients. Drivers should not be qualified if they have symptomatic congestive cardiac function. If they are asymptomatic with an EF of ≤ 50 percent but with either sustained or nonsustained ventricular tachycardia or symptomatic palpitations, they should not be qualified. Drivers can be considered for certification after disqualification if symptoms resolve, they do not have ventricular arrhythmia, and the EF improves to ≥ 40 percent. If certified, these drivers should be evaluated annually with echocardiography and Holter monitoring.

Cardiac Arrhythmias, Pacemakers, and Implantable Defibrillators

Arrhythmias are the cardiac disorders most likely to suddenly impair a driver. Driving is generally safe for most individuals with arrhythmias, but incapacitation can occur suddenly and unpredictably. The initial evaluation should include a medical history and a review of records, physical examination, and additional testing as indicated. In addition to the Advisory Panel report, one of the best reviews on the effect of arrhythmias on consciousness and the impact on public safety is by the AHA and the North American Society of Pacing and Electrophysiology (NAS) [35].

Atrial fibrillation generally is seen in older patients and usually is associated with some type of cardiovascular or metabolic diseases, e.g., thyrotoxicosis. In healthy young individuals, there may be no identifiable cause. Some patients are at increased risk of stroke with atrial fibrillation; those older than 65 year, a history of prior stroke, systemic embolism or transient ischemic attack, diabetes, hypertension, left ventricular EF < 40 percent, congestive heart failure, or left atrial size ≥ 50 mm. These patients are generally anticoagulated. Many of those drivers at risk for stroke will be disqualified for other cardiac reasons, but if not, they should be adequately anticoagulated for at least 1 month and be monitored monthly by INR, with annual re-certification. Their rate and rhythm should be adequately controlled, determined preferably by a cardiologist. If the fibrillation occurs following thoracic surgery, the drivers should also be controlled on anticoagulants for at least 1 month and be followed monthly by INR, with clearance by a cardiologist. Re-certification should be annually. Drivers with Wolf-Parkinson-White syndrome and atrial fibrillation should not be medically qualified.

In general, atrial flutter should be handled in the same manner as atrial fibrillation. If isthmus ablation is performed, the driver can return to work at least 1 month after the procedure provided the arrhythmia is successfully treated. Clearance should be by an electrophysiologist, with annual re-certification.

Drivers with multifocal atrial tachycardia can be medically qualified provided they are asymptomatic or the symptoms are controlled and the multifocal atrial tachycardia is not associated with another condition that is disqualifying such as severe pulmonary disease. Re-certification should be annual.

Ventricular arrhythmias carry a higher risk of sudden incapacitation and may be the cause of the majority of sudden cardiac deaths. Drivers with CHD and sustained ventricular tachycardia, nonsustained ventricular tachycardia (NSVT) with an EF < 40 percent, or symptomatic NSVT with an EF of ≥ 40 percent should not be certified. If the driver has NSVT with an EF ≥ 40 percent and is currently asymptomatic, he or she can be certified at least 1 month after successful drug or other treatment, with clearance by a cardiologist. Re-certification should be annual, with examination by a cardiologist.

With a diagnosis of dilated cardiomyopathy, the driver should not be certified if sustained ventricular tachycardia, NSVT with an EF ≤ 40 percent, or episodes of syncope or near syncope occur.

Drivers with long QT interval syndrome or Brugada syndrome should not be medically certified. Bundle branch block can progress, leading to third-degree heart block. Drivers who are symptomatic should not be certified. If the individual is asymptomatic and the risk from any underlying heart disease is acceptable, he or she can be certified for up to 2 years. If the driver is currently under treatment for a disease that has been symptomatic, has no underlying cardiac disease, and is cleared by a cardiologist, he or she can be certified but should be re-certified annually.

With sinus node dysfunction or atrioventricular block, the driver should not be certified until at least 1 month after pacemaker insertion, provided that underlying heart disease is not disqualifying. Re-certification should be annual, with documented pacemaker checks.

Drivers with symptoms from neurocardiogenic syncope or hypersensitive carotid sinus with syncope should not be certified unless a pacemaker has been inserted and after a 3-month wait. This wait is recommended as the cardioinhibitory (slowing of heart rate) will be treated by the pacemaker while the pacemaker may not entirely correct the vasodepressor (drop in BP) component of the syndrome. Absence of symptom recurrence and documentation of correct pacemaker function should be required prior to certification. Re-certification should be annual, with pacemaker checks and no recurrence of symptoms.

Implantable cardioverter defibrillators (ICDs) are now increasingly being used in patients for both primary and secondary prevention. They do not prevent the arrhythmias but attempt to terminate the arrhythmia once it occurs. After a ventricular arrhythmia occurs, it may take 20 seconds for an ICD to discharge; during this time, a driver may lose consciousness. Drivers who have had an ICD implanted after cardiac arrest or hemodynamically significant ventricular tachycardia should not be certified. Neither should drivers where the ICD is implanted because they are felt to have sufficiently high risk of significant arrhythmias.

Although the regulations clearly state that a driver with a cardiovascular condition that may be accompanied by syncope should not be qualified to drive, the Cardiovascular Advisory Panel did not provide specific guidance on a driver who experienced a single episode of syncope. In many cases, the etiology of the event will remain unknown. Some recommend that for drivers in whom a clearly identified, nonrecurring cause can be shown, i.e., fainting from the sight of blood, prolonged standing, or fear, there be no restriction. Yet for those in whom the cause is not so obvious, further testing should be done [36]. This may include evaluations by neurologists or cardiologists. One study reviewed the approaches of arrhythmia specialists in nine countries on determining when an individual could return safely to driving [37] and found that the majority used the tilt-table test to substantiate the diagnosis of vasovagal syncope yet overused it to evaluate treatment efficiency. Participants in this study also suggested that syncope that occurred in a sitting position should be more of a concern than if it occurred in a standing position. The average suggested wait was a minimum of 2 months after successful treatment, with a range of no restriction to never returning the individual to driving. Almost all would be more conservative when dealing with a commercial driver. Tilt-table testing also is recommended by the ACC for patients in high-risk settings who either have no evidence of structural heart disease to explain the syncopal event or in whom a structural abnormality is present but not responsible for the syncope [38]. The ACC acknowledges that there is a reasonable difference of opinion on the use of the tilt-table test to assess therapy in neurally mediated syncope. Another report from the AHA/NAS points out that the use of tilt-table testing for neurally mediated syncope or presyncopal episodes is controversial [35]. Many states also have guidelines on driving restriction for individuals who have had nonseizure-related loss of consciousness. These range from 4.3 ± 4.9 (SD) months, and as demonstrated by other studies, many physicians either misunderstand or are unaware of these guidelines [39].

Congenital Heart Disease

Most drivers with symptom-limiting congenital heart disease will select themselves out of the commercial driver pool. With improvements in medical and surgical treatment, the examiner may see an increasing number of drivers with congenital heart disease. The decision to qualify should be based on the specific diagnosis, current symptoms, and the natural history of the disease, including early and late complications. The evaluation should include a medical history and a complete review of all pertinent medical records, a complete history and physical examination, a chest x-ray, and a comprehensive 2-dimensional Doppler echocardiogram. In drivers in whom cardiac arrhythmias are a concern, ambulatory monitoring at rest and during exercise should be done. In some cases, an ETT also would be useful. For drivers who had recently undergone surgery, at least a 3-month wait and clearance by a cardiologist knowledgeable in adult congenital heart disease is recommended. Drivers with congenital heart disease, whether having undergone surgical repair or followed medically, should be re-certified annually with evaluation by a cardiologist knowledgeable in adult congenital heart disease. For recommendations on specific conditions, refer to the Advisory Panel Guidelines.

Vascular Disease

The presence of associated coronary artery or cerebrovascular disease should be excluded in a driver with a history of vascular disease.

Abdominal aortic aneurysms > 5 cm in diameter carry a significant risk of rupture and mortality. The Advisory Panel recommends that all abdominal aortic aneurysms > 5 cm should be disqualifying. If it is decided that a surgical approach is not indicated, this should not constitute a clearance to drive commercial vehicles. If an aneurysm is larger than 4 cm, it should be evaluated by a vascular specialist prior to certification. If the driver is symptomatic or surgery is planned, even those drivers with abdominal aortic aneurysms between 4 and 5 cm should not be medically qualified. If surgery is not planned and there are no symptoms, the driver could be qualified annually and the size of the aneurysm followed by ultrasound. Drivers with aneurysms of the thoracic aorta should be disqualified if the aneurysm diameter is > 3.5 cm.

Drivers who have undergone surgery for repair of abdominal aortic aneurysm, thoracic aortic aneurysm, or aneurysm of another vessel should not be cleared for commercial driving for at least 3 months and should obtain clearance from a cardiovascular specialist.

Peripheral vascular disease may present with intermittent claudication. If there are no other disqualifying cardiovascular conditions, the driver can be certified but should be re-certified annually. It is recommended that the driver with pain at rest be disqualified from operating commercial vehicles. There should be at least a 3-month wait after surgery or angioplasty for peripheral vascular disease, and these drivers should also be recertified annually.

Deep venous thrombosis (DVT) can result in local complications as well as pulmonary emboli, a cause of sudden incapacitation. DVTs should be disqualifying until the driver is adequately treated. This includes no residual acute DVT, and if on Coumadin, regulated for at least 1 month, with the INR monitored at least monthly.

If there were pulmonary emboli, drivers should not be certified for at least 3 months from a pulmonary embolus. They should be on appropriate long-term therapy, and if Coumadin is used, the dosage should be regulated for at least 1 month, with follow-up INR at least monthly. These drivers should be re-certified as least annually.

The Advisory Panel recommended that the Coumadin dosage be regulated for at least 1 month prior to returning to commercial driving, not just on the medication for 1 month. In July 1996, the FHWA responded to the question of whether warfarin is an automatic disqualifier by issuing recommendations on the use of anticoagulants in commercial drivers. They stated that the use of warfarin should be one factor in deciding whether an individual can operate a commercial motor vehicle safely. The following recommendations for evaluating a driver on anticoagulants also were issued by the FHWA at that time. These may be modified to be consistent with the new guidelines.

1. Warfarin is a medical treatment that can improve the health and safety of a driver by its use and should not be automatically disqualifying. The emphasis should be on the underlying medical condition and the general health of the driver.

2. The examiner is responsible for making the decision and should consult with other physicians who have been treating the driver.

3. The INR should be used to monitor the effect of warfarin.

4. The driver on warfarin should be educated about the interaction of warfarin and other medications and about the increased risk of bleeding with trauma. He or she also should be counseled on the need for regular monitoring.

5. Because of increased sensitivity to warfarin and the risk for significant bleeding, careful consideration should be given prior to qualifying drivers using warfarin who are older than 65 years.

6. Drivers on warfarin with cerebrovascular disease are not recommended to be medically qualified due to the increased risk of intracranial hemorrhage with resulting sudden loss of consciousness.

7. Individuals should not be qualified during the first 3 months of treatment because the risk of side effects is highest during this period.

8. Individuals qualified under 49 CFR 391.41 and on warfarin should be examined yearly to monitor both the effect of warfarin and the underlying disease process.

These recommendations are likely to be reviewed in light of the new cardiovascular guidelines.

Varicose veins and superficial thrombophlebitis do not carry a significant risk of embolism. Individuals with these problems can be medically qualified if no other disqualifying abnormalities are found.

Heart Transplantation

Commercial drivers who have had a heart transplantation and want to return to work can be considered after a 1-year wait. They should be asymptomatic, cleared by a cardiologist, and stable on medications. In addition, there should be no signs of rejection. Drivers should be re-certified every 6 months after an evaluation by a cardiologist.

Cardiovascular Medications

This area is not covered in the current guidelines but the medical examiner must still review medications and any potential side effects. Reviewing the medication can also provide the examiner with information on a diagnosis that may not have been identified on the history questions. When it is discovered that a driver is on a cardiovascular medication, two main issues need to be addressed. First, what condition is the medication treating, and, second, are there significant side effects from the medication? Frequently, an individual will deny medical problems, and when the use of a medication is discovered, he or she will explain that because of the medication, he or she no longer has the medical problem.

Some of the side effects that should be addressed by an examiner performing a commercial driver medical examination are somnolence, fatigue, impaired judgment, impaired reflexes, neurologic dysfunction, and orthostatic changes.

Conclusion

It is important not to evaluate the cardiovascular condition in isolation. A driver with multiple medical problems, all with borderline control, may be at greater risk than a driver with only one condition at the same level of stability.

The most important aspect of evaluating a cardiac patient's ability to operate a commercial motor vehicle safely is his or her underlying cardiac status. Will such a driver's heart allow him or her to perform the tasks required safely without ischemia or arrhythmia? Is the driver likely to have his or her level of alertness impaired owing to cardiac conditions or medications? Assessment of most drivers with cardiac disease should include an ECG, echocardiogram, and ETT and, depending on the diagnosis, 24-hour ambulatory monitoring. In select cases, cardiac catheterization or electrophysiologic studies may be indicated.

References

1. National Transportation Safety Board. *Fatigue, Alcohol, Other Drugs and Medical Factors in Fatal-to-Driver Heavy Truck Crashes.* PB90-917992, NTSB/SS-90/01. Washington: NTSB, 1990.
2. Dionne G, Desjarding D, Laberge-Nadeau C, Maaz U. Medical conditions, risk exposure, and truck drivers' accidents: An analysis with count data regression models. *Accid Anal Prev* 1995;27:295–305.
3. Guibert R, Duarte-Franco E, Ciampi A, et al. Medical conditions and the risk of motor vehicle crashes in men. *Arch Fam Med* 1998;7:554–558.
4. Medgyesi M, Koch D. Medical impairments to driving: Cardiovascular disease, in 39th Annual Proceedings of the Association for the Advancement of Automotive Medicine, October 1995:483–499.
5. Stewart RB, Moore MT, Marks RG, et al. *Driving Cessation and Accidents in the Elderly: An Analysis of Symptoms, Diseases, Cognitive Dysfunction and Medications.* New York: AAA Foundation for Traffic Safety, 1993.
6. Diller E, Cook L, Leonard D, et al. Evaluating drivers with medical conditions in Utah 1992–1996. NHSTA technical reports, contract DTNH22-96-H-59017, 1996.
7. Bellet S, Roman L, Kostis J, Slater A. Continuous electrocardiographic monitoring during automobile driving: Studies in normal subjects and patients with coronary disease. *Am J Cardiol* 1968;22:856–862.
8. Cocco G, Iselin HU. Cardiac risk of speed traps. *Clin Cardiol* 1992;15:441–444.
9. Dhala A, Bremner S, Blanck Z, et al. Impairment of driving abilities in patients with supraventricular tachycardia. *Am J Cardiol* 1995;75:516–518.
10. Belkic K, Savic C, Theorell T, et al. Mechanisms of cardiac risk among professional drivers. *Scand J Work Environ Health* 1994;20:73–86.

11. King D, Benbow SJ, Barrett JA. The law and medical fitness to drive: A study of doctor's knowledge. *Prostgrad Med J* 1992;68:624–628.

12. U.S. Department of Transportation, Federal Highway Administration. *Conference on Cardiac Disorders and Commercial Drivers.* Publication No. FHWA-MC-88-040. Washington: U.S. DOT, Federal Highway Administration, Office of Motor Carriers, 1987.

13. Blumenthal R, Braunstein J, Connolly H, Epstein A, Gersh BJ, Wittels EH. *Cardiovascular Advisory Panel Guidelines for the Medical Examination of Commercial Motor Vehicle Drivers.* FMCSA-MCP-02-002. Washington: U.S. Department of Transportation, Federal Motor Carrier Safety Administration, October 2002.

14. Canadian Medical Society. Determining Medical Fitness to Drive: A Guide for Physicians, 6th ed. Ottawa, Ontario: Canadian Medical Society, 2000. *http://www.cma.ca.* Accessed March 14, 2003.

15. Australasian Faculty of Occupational Medicine. *Medical Examinations of Commercial Vehicle Drivers.* Prepared for the National Road Transport Commission and the Federal Office of Road Safety, Australia, 1999. *http://www.nrtc.gov.au/publications/medstand .asp?lo=public.* Accessed March 14, 2003.

16. Drivers Medical Group. *For Medical Practitioners: At a Glance Guide to the Current Medical Standards of Fitness to Drive.* Swansea, England: Driver and Vehicle Licensing Agency, 1999. *http://www.dvla.gov.uk/ at_a_glance/content.htm.* Accessed March 14, 2003.

17. The Sixth Report of the Joint National Committee on the Prevention, Detection, Evaluation and Treatment of High Blood Pressure. *Arch Intern Med* 1997;157:2413–2446.

18. Poulter N, Marmot MG. Hypertension and the probability of an incapacitating event over a defined period: Impact of treatment. *Eur Heart J* 1992;13(suppl H):39–44.

19. Canadian Cardiovascular Society. Assessment of the cardiac patient for fitness to drive. *Can J Cardiol* 1992;8:406–412.

20. Anonymous. Assessment of the cardiac patient for fitness to drive: 1996 update. *Can J Cardiol* 1996;12(11):1164–1170, 1175–1182.

21. Petch MC. Driving and heart disease. *Eur Heart J* 1998;19:1165–1177.

22. Antecol DH, Roberts WC. Sudden death behind the wheel from natural disease in drivers of four-wheeled motorized vehicles. *Am J Cardiol* 1990;66:1329–1335.

23. Anderson MA, Camm AJ. Legal and ethical aspects of driving and working in patients with an implantable cardioverter defibrillator. *Am Heart J* 1994;127:1185–1193.24.

24. Rosengren A, Anderson K, Wilhelmsen L. Risk of coronary heart disease in middle-aged male bus and tram drivers compared to men in other occupations: A prospective study. *Int J Epidemiol* 1991;20: 82–87.

25. Executive Summary of the Third Report of the National Cholesterol Education Program (NCEP) Expert Panel on the Detection, Evaluation, and Treatment of High Blood Cholesterol in Adults (Adult Treatment Panel III) *http://www.nhlbi.nih.gov/guidelines/cholesterol/atp_iii.htm*. Accessed March 14, 2003.

26. Grundy SM, Pasternak R, Greenland P, et al. Assessment of cardiovascular risk by use of multiple risk factor assessment equations: A statement for healthcare professionals from the American Heart Association. *Circulation* 1999;100:1481–1492.

27. Snader CD, Marwick TH, Pashkow FJ, et al. Importance of estimated functional capacity as a predictor of all-cause mortality among patients referred for exercise thallium single-photon emission computed tomography: Report of 3400 patients from a single center. *J Am Coll Cardiol* 1997;30:641–648.

28. Beller GA. Assessing prognosis by means of radionuclide perfusion imaging: What technique and which variables should be used? *J Am Coll Cardiol* 1998;31:1286–1290.

29. Multicenter Postinfarction Research Group. Risk stratification and survival after myocardial infarction. *N Engl J Med* 1983;309:331–336.

30. *U.S. Preventive Services Task Force (USPSTF) in the Guide to Clinical Preventive Services*, 2nd ed. Baltimore: Williams & Wilkins, 1996.

31. The Joint European Society/American College of Cardiology Committee. Myocardial infarction redefined: A consensus document of the Joint European Society of Cardiology/American College of Cardiology Committee for the redefinition of myocardial infarction. *Eur Heart J* 2000;21:1502–1513.

32. Meier MA, Al-Badr WH, Cooper JV, Kline-Rogers EM, Smith DE, Eagle KA, Mehta RH. The new definition of myocardial infarction: Diagnostic and prognostic implications in patients with acute coronary syndromes. *Arch Intern Med* 2002;162:1585–1589.

33. Bonow RO, ACC/AHA Task Force Report. Guidelines for the management of patients with valvular heart disease. *J Am Coll Cardiol* 1998;32:1486–1588.

34. Amato MCM, Moffa PJ, Werner KE, Ramires JA. Treatment decision in asymptomatic aortic valve stenosis: Role of exercise testing. *Heart* 2001;86:381–386.

35. Epstein AE, Miles WM, Benditt DG, et al. Personal and public safety issues related to arrhythmias that may affect consciousness: Implications for regulation and physician recommendations. *Circulation* 1996;94:1147–1166.

36. Linzer M, Yang EH, Estes NAM, et al. Diagnosing syncope: I. Value of history, physical examination and electrocardiography. *Ann Intern Med* 1997;126:989–996.

37. Lurie KG, Iskos D, Sakaguchi S, et al. Resumption of motor vehicle operations in vasovagal fainters. *Am J Cardiol* 1999;83:604–606.
38. Benditt DG, Ferguson DW, Grubb BP, et al. ACC expert consensus document: Tilt-table testing for assessing syncope. *J Am Coll Cardiol* 1996;28:263–275.
39. Strickberger SA, Cantilloon CO, Friedman PL. When should patients with lethal ventricular arrhythmia resume driving? An analysis of state regulation and physician practices. *Ann Intern Med* 1991;115:560–563.

Additional References

Laberge-Nadeau C, Dione G, Maag D, et al. Medical conditions and the severity of commercial motor vehicle drivers' road accidents. *Accid Anal Prev* 1996;28(1):43–51.

Larsen GC, Stupey MR, Walance CG, et al. Recurrent cardiac events in survivors of ventricular fibrillation or tachycardia: Implications for driving restrictions. *JAMA* 1994;271:1335–1339.

Levine M, Hirsch J, Landefeld S, Raskob G. Hemorrhagic complications of anticoagulant treatment. *Chest* 1992;102:352S–363S.

Lown B. Management of patients at high risk of sudden cardiac death. *Am Heart J* 1982;103:689–697.

Myerburg RJ, Kessler KM, Castellanos A. Sudden cardiac death: Structure, function and time-dependence of risk. *Circulation* 1992;85(suppl 1):2–10.

Petch M, Irvine J. Cardiovascular disorders and vocational driving. *Practitioner* 1995;239:37–39.

Pryor DB, Bruce RA, Chaitman BR, et al. Task force I: Determination of prognosis in patients with ischemic heart disease. *J Am Coll Cardiol* 1989;14:1016–1025.

Severi S, Michelassi C. Prognostic impact of stress testing in coronary artery disease. *Circulation* 1991;83(suppl 3):82–88.

Shephard RJ. Cardiovascular risk and truck driving. *J Cardiopulm Rehabil* 1986;6:260–262.

Shephard RJ. The cardiac patient and driving: The Ontario experience. In: *Conference on Cardiac Disorders and Commercial Drivers*. Baltimore: U.S. Department of Transportation, Federal Highway Administration, 1987:85–94.

Wielgosz AT, Azad N. Effects of cardiovascular disease on driving tasks. *Clin Geriatr Med* 1993;9:341–348.

5

Pulmonary Disorders

NATALIE P. HARTENBAUM, MD, MPH

The respiratory system is responsible for providing adequate oxygen to the tissues and removing carbon dioxide from the bloodstream. The brain and heart are particularly sensitive to oxygen deprivation. Acute or chronic abnormalities in oxygen content or carrying capacity of the blood may result either directly or indirectly in confusion, dizziness, or loss of consciousness.

Respiratory problems are not as likely as cardiac or neurologic dysfunction to suddenly incapacitate a driver. As pulmonary function declines, it becomes more difficult for a driver to perform required tasks aside from driving. It is estimated that truck driving itself requires 3.0 metabolic equivalents [METs, defined as the energy demand in liters of oxygen consumption per minute of basal oxygen consumption (3.5 mL/kg per minute)], whereas lifting and carrying 60 to 80 lb requires 7.5 METs [1]. With mild impairment, pulmonary function test (PFT) abnormalities may not correlate well with complaints of dyspnea. As respiratory function declines, there is a direct correlation. The more abnormal the PFT, the less likely it is that the individual will be able to work as a commercial driver.

Sleep apnea, and its resulting daytime somnolence or decreased alertness, has been recognized as a potential cause of motor vehicle accidents. The new Medical Examination Reporting Form includes a question on sleep apnea and other sleep disorders, requiring drivers to indicate whether they have a "sleep disorder, pauses in breathing while sleeping, daytime sleepiness, loud snoring."

Many medications used to treat respiratory conditions such as allergies or cough have potentially serious side effects. These side effects must be taken into account during the decision-making process.

The standard addressing respiratory function [49 CFR 391.41(b)(5)] states that

A person is physically qualified to drive a commercial motor vehicle if that person: (5) Has no established medical history or clinical diagnosis of a respiratory dysfunction likely to interfere with his/her ability to control and drive a motor vehicle safely.

The intent of the Federal Motor Carrier Safety Administration (FMCSA) regarding pulmonary disqualification is widely open to interpretation. The medical advisory criteria explain that impairment in respiratory function, especially when there is greater oxygen demand, as in emergency situations, may be "detrimental to safe driving." Sleep apnea is now included as one of the conditions that may interfere with adequate respiratory function. The medical examiner is advised to refer to a specialist if any abnormality that may interfere with safe operation of the commercial motor vehicle is detected. If the driver is on anticoagulation therapy for deep venous thrombosis or pulmonary embolus, they can be qualified once the lower extremity vascular studies are normal and the optimal dose of anticoagulation has been reached. The advisory criteria refer the driver to the Conference on Pulmonary/Respiratory Disorders and Commercial Drivers [2]. The cardiac advisory criteria also offer that the examiner may contact the Federal Motor Carrier Safety Administration (FMCSA) at 202-366-1790 for additional information on qualifying drivers on Coumadin. The guidance (Figure 5-1) on Coumadin was issued in response to questions on the use of anticoagulants but will be updated with issuance of the new cardiovascular guidelines.

Recommendations

The qualification recommendations in the remainder of this chapter are from the FHWA pulmonary conference [2], except where indicated. Additional information on some conditions is included, and the reference source noted.

Evaluation

In screening drivers for pulmonary disease, questions that should be asked include

Do you smoke? If so, how much? For how many years?

Do you feel short of breath with activity or while driving?

Do you cough? If so, is your cough productive of sputum?

Figure 5-1. The commercial driver on Coumadin

Part 391 of the Federal Motor Carrier Safety Regulations has been designed to protect both the health and safety of the driver and the general public. As drivers age and as the indications for anticoagulation with Coumadin increase, it is important to review the effect of Coumadin on the commercial driver's health and risk to the general public from commercial drivers on Coumadin. Based on reviews of the medical literature, regulations form other regulatory agencies, and the policies of other countries, the following recommendations have been reached.

1. Coumadin is a medical treatment which can improve the health and safety of the driver and should not, by its use, medically disqualify the commercial driver. The emphasis should be on the underlying medical condition(s) which require treatment and the general health of the driver.

2. The medical examiner responsible for making the qualification determination should confer with other doctors who have treated the driver.

3. The International Normalized Ratio (INR) is now the best available methods to monitor the anticoagulant effect of Coumadin. It also allows results from different laboratories to be compared. This method is strongly recommended for monitoring the effect of Coumadin.

4. A driver on Coumadin should be educated about the potential interaction of Coumadin with other medications and diet, the increase risk of bleeding with trauma and the need for regular monitoring of Coumadin's effect.

5. The medical certification of commercial drivers on Coumadin and over age 65 should receive careful consideration because of the increased sensitivity to Coumadin and the risk for significant bleeding.

6. The medical certification of commercial drivers with cerebrovascular disease and who are on Coumadin is not recommended because of the increased risk of intracranial hemorrhage with sudden loss of consciousness.

7. An individual should not be medically certified during the first 3 months on Coumadin because the major risk from side effects of Coumadin occur within these first months on treatment.

8. An individual should have a physical examination every year under section 391.43, instead of every 2 years, because of the need to monitor closely both the effect of Coumadin and the underlying medical condition(s).

Revised: April 1996
US Department of Transportation
Federal Highway Administration

Do you have tightness in your chest during exercise or at rest?

Do you snore? If so, do you feel sleepy during the day?

Do you wheeze?

In addition to obvious signs of shortness of breath (e.g., a patient becomes short of breath just getting onto the examining table), other physical signs of pulmonary disease may include clubbing; cyanosis; slowing of expiration; tachypnea at rest; diffuse rhonchi, wheezes, or rales; decreased or absent breath sounds; pleural rubs; significant kyphosis; or use of accessory muscles of ventilation at rest.

Pulmonary Function Tests (PFTs). Participants in the Pulmonary/ Respiratory Disorders Conference recommended PFTs as an integral part of lung function evaluation. They suggest PFTs for any driver with a history of lung disease or symptoms of shortness of breath, cough, chest tightness, or wheezing. PFTs also are recommended for all cigarette smokers older than 35 years. While this may identify all drivers with suboptimal lung function, the cost and number of normal tests will make this cost-prohibitive. However, many of the drivers with lung function below the levels recommended likely will have some physical signs to suggest impairment.

Recommendations from the report for certification are based on PFTs where indicated. For drivers who have normal PFTs, no further evaluation is needed. For drivers with obstructive disease, if the PFTs are abnormal, forced expiratory volume in 1 second (FEV_1) < 65% of predicted, forced vital capacity (FVC) < 60% of predicted, or FEV_1/FVC ratio < 65%, arterial blood gases (ABGs) or pulse oximetry was recommended. The criterion for performing ABGs or pulse oximetry in patients with restrictive diseases is an FVC < 60% of predicted. If the screening pulse oximetry is < 92%, then ABGs should be reviewed. A partial pressure of arterial oxygen (PaO_2) of < 65 mm Hg or a partial pressure of carbon dioxide ($PaCO_2$) of > 45 mm Hg should cause the driver to not be medically qualified. One method of evaluating the efficiency of gas exchange is through diffusing lung capacity of carbon monoxide(DL_{CO}). If the results here are < 60% of predicted, further studies also should be obtained.

Infectious Diseases

Acute respiratory infections such as influenza, bronchitis, or the common cold generally will not have long-term safety implications. During an acute infection, the symptoms may interfere with the ability to perform heavy work and with alertness. Regulating these short-term diseases is not practical. Pneumonia should preclude commercial driving until the infection has been adequately treated.

The respiratory status of individuals with underlying chronic but stable conditions such as asthma or chronic bronchitis may decompensate significantly with respiratory infections or influenza. When evaluating drivers with chronic pulmonary disorders, it is important to determine whether their status may change significantly with acute exacerbations. Drivers who are able to do so may take sick or vacation time, but the long-haul trucker may be at the other end of the United States when symptoms occur and may have no choice but to continue working. Medications may be taken to treat the congestion, runny nose, or cough, but some can have potentially dangerous side effects. All drivers should be warned at the time of the medical evaluation to exercise caution when using any medication while working, including those available over the counter.

Infection and hemoptysis are concerns in individuals with bronchiectasis, a disease characterized by inflammatory destruction of the bronchioles. For them, pulmonary function should be evaluated, and drivers not meeting the criteria listed earlier should not be qualified. Drivers with a recent episode of hemoptysis of >250 mL or with recurrent exacerbations also should be disqualified.

Clinical manifestation of tuberculosis can range from a positive tuberculin test to advanced disease. If chest x-rays do not indicate recent infection or a change from earlier evaluations, there is no reason to deny certification. Recent tuberculin test conversion should prompt the initiation of treatment, but the driver can continue to work once treatment has been initiated. If streptomycin is required as the drug of choice, the driver should not be medically qualified until the treatment is completed because of streptomycin's effect on hearing and balance. Individuals with severe disease, as determined through PFTs and chest x-rays, or those with inadequately treated disease or chronic tuberculosis should be disqualified.

Atypical tuberculosis is generally not a contagious disease. The driver should be allowed to work if pulmonary function is adequate. If coexistent medical conditions or the infection itself causes fatigue, weakness, or other interfering symptoms, the driver should not be medically qualified.

Noninfectious Diseases

Noninfectious diseases include chest wall deformities, interstitial lung diseases, and chronic obstructive pulmonary disease (COPD). A thorough history and physical examination are essential. Lung status should be evaluated through the PFTs, chest x-rays, and ABGs, if indicated. In some patients, it may be desirable to assess O_2 saturation response to exercise. Decisions as to certification should be individualized but based on PFTs or O_2 saturation response to exercise. When exercise testing is chosen as part of the evaluation for pulmonary disease, the driver should be able to reach at least 4.3 METs. If the driver is unable to do so, or if there is a drop in O_2 saturation, he or she should not be qualified.

Many individuals with COPD will have minimal physical findings. As lung function deteriorates, work ability also declines. The risk of COPD increases with increasing years of smoking, and, therefore, PFTs were recommended for all smokers older than 35 years.

The American Medical Association (AMA) guidelines, which are now almost 2 decades old and have not been updated, based their recommendation on drivers with COPD on clinical findings, in addition to the standard physiologic studies [3]. The AMA suggested that individuals with moderate to severe respiratory impairment be restricted from commercial vehicle driving. Such impairment includes dyspnea while walking on level ground or up one flight of stairs. The FEV_1 in such individuals would be < 59% of predicted, and the FVC < 60% of predicted. More recent guidelines from the Canadian Medical Association (CMA) [4] also base recommendations on level of impairment. Drivers with COPD and no or only mild impairment would be permitted to operate commercial vehicles. The CMA defined this as dyspnea when walking quickly on level ground or when walking uphill or ability to keep pace with others of similar age and build on level ground but not on hills. The CMA also advised against permitting individuals who require oxygen to operate commercial motor vehicles.

COPD also carries the risk of cough syncope. Drivers with COPD and cough syncope should not be qualified because cough syncope can be unpredictable and incapacitating. Great Britain's Driver and Vehicle Licensing Agency (DVLA) recommended that driving cease until the driver is no longer liable to have attacks [5]. There were few other DVLA recommendations on the medical qualification of commercial drivers with pulmonary diseases. In their *Guide to Medical Standards,* the DVLA notes that COPD should be disqualifying only if the driver has experienced loss of consciousness during an exacerbation.

Cystic fibrosis may present with end-stage COPD. In the past, many cystic fibrosis patients did not survive into adulthood. Now, however, with numerous medical advances, many do, and those who wish to enter the commercial driver pool should be evaluated with the same criteria as others with COPD. Depending on the driver's current status, evaluation more frequently than every 2 years may be desirable.

A pneumothorax may be idiopathic or due to trauma. Traumatic pneumothoraces often are easily treated and unlikely to recur. In a commercial driver, complete resolution should be documented by chest x-ray, and if no other abnormalities are present, the driver may be qualified. There is a 25% risk of recurrence of spontaneous pneumothoraces in the first 2 years, increasing to 85% in individuals with a history of three prior spontaneous pneumothoraces. Spontaneous pneumothoraces usually are associated with underlying lung disease. Drivers with a history of two or more spontaneous pneumothoraces on the same side should not be qualified. After successful pleurodesis, a driver with recurrent pneumothoraces can be qualified if other pulmonary parameters are within acceptable ranges. Drivers with a single spontaneous pneumothorax and no associated pulmonary disease can be qualified if they have no chest pain or shortness of breath and if resolution of the pneumothorax has been confirmed.

Allergies

Allergies are very common and, in and of themselves, are unlikely to cause a problem for commercial drivers. Studies have evaluated the effect of antihistamines on driving and have concluded that they do have a significant effect on performance [6,7]. Some states have laws against driving under the influence of any agent that impairs performance, including antihistamines [8]. Drivers with allergic rhinitis should be advised to use the nonsedating antihistamines or local steroid sprays. Those with severe symptoms, such as uncontrollable sneezing or impaired vision due to ophthalmic involvement, should refrain temporarily from driving.

Asthmatics can be certified, but their pulmonary function should meet the recommended criteria. Some tasks associated with commercial driving may exacerbate asthma, such as exposure to nonspecific irritants or cold temperatures. Recurrent hospitalizations or a frequent need for high-dose steroids should prompt further evaluation. If a driver is severely symptomatic, or if there is significant pulmonary impairment ($FEV_1 < 65\%$ or $PaO_2 < 65$ mm Hg) that cannot be reversed by treatment, the driver should not be medically qualified. Great Britain's DVLA indicates that unless asthma is associated with sudden loss of consciousness during an attack, there is no reason to restrict commercial driving.

Hypersensitivity pneumonitis can be associated with dyspnea, cough, or fever. However, drivers with hypersensitivity pneumonitis can be qualified, but they should avoid the causative agent, and, if possible, they should take preventive precautions.

Drivers with a history of allergy to stinging insects not only may be incapacitated from a sting but also may panic at the sight of an insect. Immunotherapy may be indicated depending on the severity of reactions, and injectable epinephrine must be available.

Hereditary or acquired angioedema can be controlled with treatment, and if it is, commercial driving is acceptable. Recurrent episodes of idiopathic anaphylaxis may be difficult to control. If such episodes are due to a recognized allergen that can be avoided, or if the symptoms can be managed, driver qualification may be acceptable. When such a driver is unable to prevent the sudden onset of dyspnea or loss of consciousness, he or she should be medically disqualified.

Secondary Pulmonary Conditions

Pneumonectomy is usually done to remove a cancerous growth; it also may be performed to remove a diseased portion of tissue in otherwise healthy lungs. Certification of drivers who have undergone pneumonectomy should be based on the underlying disease process and pulmonary function. Most individuals without other pulmonary disease will do well after surgery. If such individuals meet PFT and ABG criteria, they should be medically qualified.

A *tracheostomy* does not itself present a danger, but as in several other situations, concern focuses on the disease that necessitated the procedure. When the tracheostomy is done because of surgery for cancer of the head or neck, the functional status and progression of the disease should guide the driver qualification decision. If the tracheostomy was performed because of acute but reversible respiratory disease, the stoma usually is permitted to heal once the acute episode has resolved. Occasionally, sleep apnea is treated with a tracheostomy, and in such a circumstance, the sleep apnea should be controlled, as described below, prior to driver qualification.

Long-haul drivers who go for long periods of time without changing position may be at risk for *deep venous thrombosis* (DVT) and possible resulting *pulmonary embolism* (PE), with shortness of breath, cardiac insufficiency, or collapse. An increased risk of recurrence may exist for several months after the initial incident. One month of anticoagulation treatment is recommended prior to returning to work, and resolution of the thrombus or embolus should be confirmed by Doppler study, impedance plethysmography, venography, or other methods.

In 1992, at the time of the pulmonary conference, the FHWA recommended against the use of oral anticoagulants in commercial drivers. Due in part to the recommendations of the pulmonary task force and to the ability of lower doses of sodium warfarin (Coumadin) to decrease the risk of hemorrhage while still preventing PE and DVT, revised Medical Advisory Criteria were issued. Additional guidance was prepared for the examiner in 1996 (see Figure 5-1). The pulmonary conference participants believed that drivers using warfarin should be permitted to be certified but that their prothrombin time (PT) should be maintained between 1.2 and 1.5, and it was further recommended that the PT be monitored every 2 weeks. The examiner and the driver's treating physician should discuss the individual case, and both should concur that the driver in question could safely be medically qualified. Drivers returning to work after DVT should be counseled about the importance of frequent position changes and should be encouraged to stop the truck and walk hourly if possible.

Despite symptoms, both pulmonary and constitutional, that may occur with either primary or secondary *lung carcinoma*, some of these individuals can be qualified as commercial drivers. Individuals not currently receiving treatment who do not have severe cough, dyspnea, or brain involvement and have a $PaO_2 > 65$ mm Hg could be medically qualified. However, they should be reevaluated every 3 months for 2 years and then yearly for 5 years. If such individuals are currently receiving treatment, have no severe side effects of the treatment such as nausea, vomiting, or weakness, and meet other criteria, they should be medically qualified but evaluated monthly. Great Britain's DVLA recommends a 2-year cessation from commercial driving after treatment for carcinoma of the lung. Such drivers also should be free from evidence of cerebral metastasis before resuming driving.

Cor pulmonale is right ventricular dysfunction caused by pulmonary hypertension, usually as a result of pulmonary disease. Pulmonary hypertension also can be caused by left ventricular dysfunction. Patients with pulmonary hypertension or cor pulmonale may experience shortness of breath, chest pain, dizziness, or syncope. Abnormalities such as distended neck veins, liver enlargement, or peripheral edema may be found on physical examination. Cardiac findings may include a P_2, right-sided S_3, or murmur of tricuspid insufficiency. Electrocardiographic or chest x-ray abnormalities are also possible, but the diagnosis is confirmed by right heart catheterization. Vasodilators may be used to treat this disease, and they can produce hypotension, dizziness, or syncope. ABG criteria must be met for such a driver to be qualified. The driver also should be free from dyspnea at rest, dizziness, or hypotension.

After *lung transplantation,* most patients will return to adequate pulmonary function within 3 to 6 months. Return of cardiac function to normal generally is not seen in heart-lung transplant patients, and maximal O_2 response to exercise usually is impaired. If such a driver is able to return to work, his or her status should be evaluated by the standard methods. The medications used to prevent rejection, such as cyclosporine, prednisone, or azathioprine, can present risks of their own. Drug levels, blood chemistries, and blood cell counts must be monitored regularly, and the driver must not miss any doses. Such drivers should limit their geographic range so that compliance with treatment and testing regimens can be met. They also should have access to nearby tertiary centers capable of handling emergencies such as rejection so that appropriate treatment can be obtained within a few hours.

Obstructive Sleep Apnea (OSA). There was very little guidance in the pulmonary/respiratory report on OSA; however, is it referenced in both the preamble to the Final Rule for the new form [9] and the advisory criteria. The new form now includes a specific question on OSA, and it is included in the advisory criteria as a respiratory condition that may "result in incapacitation." The preamble to the Final Rule of the new form includes mention of the Parent's Against Tired Truckers (PATT) recommendation that the eight-question Epworth Sleepiness Scale (ESS) be included as part of the examination. This scale, based on an individual's subjective assessment of sleepiness, can be used by examiners, but PATT's recommendation has not been adopted.

OSA may be a significant problem among commercial drivers, and it represents a significant public health hazard [10]. It is estimated to affect 5 to 10 million Americans. There is also ample evidence that drivers with sleep disorders have as much as a sevenfold increased risk of accidents [11–15]. It has been estimated that 1% to 3% of U.S. motor vehicle crashes are caused by driver sleepiness; of those, about 3% involve commercial drivers [12].

Powell et al [16] found reaction times worse in individuals with sleep-disordered breathing than in subjects with a blood alcohol concentration of 0.057 g/dL. While drivers may be aware that they are sleepy, they may not take action to stop driving and prevent accidents.

This condition, which commonly affects obese, middle-aged males, is characterized by episodes of nocturnal asphyxia, with brief episodes of waking, snoring, and excessive daytime somnolence. The hypersomnolence that occurs during waking hours is seen most frequently during monotonous activities such as driving, thereby causing an increase in motor vehicle accidents. Drivers with sleep apnea also tend to underestimate their level of daytime sleepiness, so reliance on subjective report of somnolence may be unreliable [17]. The use of alcohol or sedatives, shift work, and sleep deprivation can further exacerbate the degree of impairment. Physical finding to suggest OSA [18] may include obesity (body mass index [BMI] > 28), increased neck circumference (≥ 16 $^1/_2$ inches), craniosynostosis, mandibular hypoplasia, and retrognathia. Other findings may include elongated soft palate and uvula, high arched palate, and enlarged tonsils.

Using the ESS (Figure 5-2) [19], studies [20–22] of drivers and workers have found scores of ≥ 10 in 17% to 26% and scores of ≥ 15 in 1.8% to 2.5%. In one large U.S. trucking company [23] using a portable monitor and a validated symptom questionnaire, 78% of the drivers had a > 5% oxygen desaturation index (ODI) ≥ 5 per hour of sleep, with 10% having an ODI of ≥ 30 per hour of sleep. There was a significant relationship between BMI and ODI in these drivers. In a project [24]

Figure 5-2. Epworth Sleepiness Scale

How likely are you to fall asleep in the following situations?

0 — would never doze

1 — slight chance of dozing

2 — moderate chance of dozing

3 — high chance of dozing

_____ Sitting and reading

_____ Watching TV

_____ Sitting, inactive in a public place (e.g., theater or meeting)

_____ As a passenger in the car for an hour without a break

_____ Lying down to rest in the afternoon when circumstances permit

_____ Sitting and talking with someone

_____ Sitting quietly after a lunch without alcohol

_____ In a car, while stopped for a few minutes in traffic

More than 10 — sleepy

More than 15 — dangerously sleepy

---

sponsored by the FMCSA and the American Transportation Research Institute of the American Trucking Association, among their sample of commercial driver's license holders, 17.6% had mild sleep apnea, 5.8% had moderate sleep apnea, and 4.7% had severe sleep apnea, a prevalence similar to the general population. The prevalence of sleep apnea depended on the relationship between age and obesity. Daytime performance depended not only on the severity of sleep apnea but also on the average duration of sleep of the driver.

Among 448 patients with OSA in one study [25], almost 9% had been involved in an automobile accident, mainly caused by falling asleep at the wheel, within the proceeding 5 years. In this group, excessive sleepiness was associated with an ESS of >11 and an Apnea/Hypopnea Index (AHI) of > 15. In another study, drivers found to have an AHI of 10 or higher had an odds ratio of 6.3 for having a traffic accident [11]. Increased risk remained even after controlling for confounders.

It can be difficult to determine which patients should undergo the expensive and not conveniently available polysomnogram. This test is considered the gold standard in the diagnosis of OSA. It simultaneously measures electroencephalography, respiration, electrocardiography, and oxygenation, assessing apneic episodes and sleep stages. One of the measures reported is the Respiratory Disturbance Index (RDI) or AHI. OSA can be classified as mild to severe based on the RDI (Figure 5-3).

A 2-step algorithm [26] utilizing nocturnal pulse oximetry and the Multivariable Apnea Prediction questionnaire [27] allowed the

Figure 5-3. Respiratory Disturbance Index

Parameter	Normal	Mild	Moderate	Severe
RDI	0–5	5–15	15–30	> 30
Lowest O_2 saturation	90–100%	80–89%	70–79%	< 70%
% of sleep with oxyhe-moglobin saturation < 90%	0–0.5	0.5–4	4–12	> 12
Number of cortical arousals/ hour sleep	0–17	17–23	23–30	> 30

researchers to stratify patients referred to a sleep disorder clinic into low- and higher-risk groups. Another method used for stratifying patients for testing was based on neck circumference and symptoms of daytime somnolence [28].

A diagnosis of OSA is made with an RDI of >5, but most of those in the mild category will neither require nor benefit from treatment. Identifying those at high risk of the long-term complications of OSA or at risk of motor vehicle accidents can be more difficult. Determining which require treatment can be controversial [29]. Some recommend treatment with continuous positive airway pressure (CPAP) with an RDI of >30, while others recommend treatment if the RDI is >20 [30].

The pulmonary conference report recommends that if there is any suspicion that sleep apnea exists, the driver should be referred for a further evaluation. The condition should be treated successfully prior to medical qualification. Treatment may consist of CPAP, uvulopalatopharyngoplasty, weight loss, and/or tracheostomy.

The conference participants recommended at least a 1-month waiting period prior to qualification for commercial driving. Some reports suggest that although symptom relief may be immediate, an actual reduction in daytime sleepiness may not occur for up to 6 weeks [31]. Of more concern for commercial drivers with sleep apnea, however, is that compliance with CPAP ranges from 75% to 85% and that skipping only one night of treatment can cause a return to pretreatment levels of sleepiness [32].

The conference participants also advised evaluation of the effectiveness of treatment through either multiple sleep-latency testing (MSLT) or polysomnographs. MSLT is able to evaluate the ease with which an individual can fall asleep during normal waking hours. Another test that is now available is the maintenance-of-wakefulness test, which measures the ability of an individual to remain awake. It is advised in the conference report that drivers with sleep apnea who are medically qualified to drive commercial motor vehicles be reevaluated annually by sleep studies or MSLT. The maintenance-of-wakefulness test may be more useful as it measures the ability to stay awake rather than how quickly an individual can fall asleep. Studies, however, have not demonstrated a relationship between sleep latency and reported accidents [33].

CMA guidelines [4] state that individuals "subject to sleep disorders cannot drive any type of motor vehicle safely." Drivers with moderate to severe OSA who are not compliant with treatment should not operate vehicles, nor should those with a high AHI, especially if right heart failure or daytime somnolence is present. The CMA suggests reassessment for compliance after 1 to 2 months.

The American Thoracic Society (ATS) [34] recognizes the importance of OSA's role in vehicle accidents and suggests use of a higher level of caution in commercial drivers. The ATS defines a high-risk individual as one who has excessive daytime sleepiness as well as a prior motor vehicle accident. The effectiveness of therapy, according to the ATS, can be judged within 2 months. Accurate assessments of risk and effectiveness of treatment still need to be developed.

Australia's National Road Transport Commission recommends that drivers with sleep apnea only be permitted to drive commercial vehicles once they are treated [35]. The commission cautions that the ability of a long-distance trucker to comply with CPAP or other treatments must be evaluated. Studies for the presence of sleep apnea and a conditional license with periodic examinations are advised for drivers with a combination of daytime sleepiness, a BMI >30, and a reddened, edematous, narrow oropharynx or a history of snoring and witnessed apnea.

Some states, such as California and Texas, do address sleep apnea in their medical criteria for drivers [15], so it is important to also be aware of both the state where you are licensed and where the driver has obtained his or her commercial driver's license.

(A complete discussion of OSA and its diagnosis, treatment, and prognosis is beyond the scope of this chapter. Please refer to the references for additional information on this medical condition.)

Pulmonary Medications

With respiratory disorders, the medications used to treat the diseases and symptoms may be more dangerous than the disease itself. The sympathomimetics elevate blood pressure and can cause rapid heart rates or arrhythmias. Some antihistamines may produce drowsiness. Narcotics in cough medication also can cause sedation. The sedating medications should be avoided for at least 12 hours prior to driving. Drivers subject to random drug and alcohol testing also should be cautioned against taking a family member's narcotic-containing cough medication. Aside from the potential consequences of driving under the influence of these medications, if a driver is subject to a random drug test and is found to be positive, some Medical Review Officers may downgrade a spousal-use opiate from positive, but most will not.

Amantadine is used for patients with influenza A and may cause confusion in the elderly. Other antimicrobials used in acute respiratory infections generally will not cause problems.

Medications used to treat tuberculosis have significant toxicity. Rifampin and ethambutol can cause confusion, dizziness, weakness, and visual disturbances. The use of streptomycin in commercial drivers should be avoided or closely monitored because it can affect balance or hearing.

Methylxanthines can cause confusion with elevated levels and should be monitored. Inhaled steroids generally will not cause problems, but oral steroids may cause confusion. Inhaled cromolyn is generally safe. A new class of asthma medications, leukotriene-receptor antagonists, may prolong the PT if used with warfarin.

Conclusion

The bottom line with pulmonary disorders and medical certification is that regardless of the disease, the decision should be based on lung function. PFTs should be obtained first, followed by ABGs or, if clinically indicated, exercise studies. In the competitive market for occupational health services, obtaining all recommended studies may be difficult and costly. There is always an examiner willing to cut costs when pushed, especially if the testing is not mandated.

Medications and accompanying side effects are relevant and should be evaluated. Awareness of the effects of sleep apnea is growing, and such effects must be addressed in evaluating the medical fitness of commercial drivers.

References

1. Harber P, Fedoruk MJ. Work placement and worker fitness: Implications of the Americans with Disabilities Act for pulmonary medicine. *Chest* 1994;105:1564–1571.
2. U.S. Department of Transportation, Federal Highway Administration. *Conference on Respiratory/Pulmonary Disorders and Commercial Drivers.* Publication No. FHWA-MC-91-004. Washington: U.S. DOT, Federal Highway Administration, Office of Motor Carriers, 1991.

3. American Medical Association. *Medical Conditions Affecting Drivers.* Chicago: AMA, 1986.

4. Canadian Medical Association. *Physicians' Guide to Driver Examination,* 6th ed. Ottawa: CMA, 2000.

5. Drivers Medical Group. *For Medical Practitioners, At-a-Glance Guide to the Current Medical Standards of Fitness to Drive.* Swansea, England: Driver and Vehicle Licensing Agency, February 2002 version. *http://www.dvla.gov.uk/at_a_glance/content.htm.* Accessed Nov. 18, 2002.

6. O'Hanlon JF, Ramaekers JG. Antihistamine effects on actual driving performance in a standard test: A summary of Dutch experience, 1989–1994. *Allergy* 1995;50:234–242.

7. Reidel WJ, Schoenmakers EAJM, O'Hanlon JF. Sedation and performance impairment with antihistamines. In: Kalinger MA, ed. *Management of Allergy in the 1990s.* Toronto: Hans Huber, 1989:38–49.

8. U.S. Department of Transportation. *Digest of State Alcohol-Related Highway Safety Legislation,* 14th ed. Washington: U.S. DOT, 1996.

9. Physical Qualification of Drivers; Medical Examination; Final rule. *Fed Reg* 2000;65(Oct. 5):59363–59380.

10. Dement WC, Mitler MM. It's time to wake up to the importance of sleep disorders. *JAMA* 1993;269:1548–1549.

11. Teran-Santos J, Jimenez-Gomez A, Cordero-Guevara J. The association between sleep apnea and the risk of traffic accidents. *N Engl J Med* 1999;340:847–851.

12. Lyznicki JM, Doege TC, Davis RM, Williams MA. Sleepiness, driving, and motor vehicle crashes. *JAMA* 1998;279:1908–1913.

13. Pack AI, Pack AM, Rodgman E, et al. Characteristics of crashes attributed to the driver having fallen asleep. *Accid Anal Prev* 1995;27:769–775.

14. Horstman S, Hess CW, Bassetti C, Gugger M, Mathis J. Sleepiness related accidents in sleep apnea patients. *Sleep* 200;23:283–289.

15. Pakola SJ, Dinges DF, Pack AI. Driving and sleepiness: Review of regulations and guidelines for commercial and noncommercial drivers with sleep apnea and narcolepsy. *Sleep* 1995;18(9):787–796.

16. Powell NB, Riley RW, Schechtman KB, Blumen MB, Dinges DF, Guilleminault C. A comparative model: Reaction time performance in sleep-disordered breathing versus alcohol-impaired controls. *Laryngoscope* 1999;109:1648–1654.

17. Engelman HM, Hirst WS, Douglas NJ. Underreporting of sleepiness and driving impairment in patients with sleep apnea/hypopnea syndrome. *J Sleep Res* 1997;6:272–275.

18. Attarian HP, Sabri AN. When to suspect obstructive sleep apnea syndrome: Symptoms may be subtle, but treatment is straightforward. *Postgrad Med* 2002;111:70–76.

19. Krieger J. Clinical approach to excessive daytime sleepiness. *Sleep* 2000;23(Suppl 4):S95–S98.

20. Benbadis SR, Perry MC, Sundstad LS, Wolgamuth BR. Prevalence of daytime sleepiness in a population of drivers. *Neurology* 1999;52:209–210.

21. Johns M, Hocking B. Daytime sleepiness and sleep habits of Australian workers. *Sleep* 1997;20:844–849.

22. Maycock G. Sleepiness and driving: The experience of UK car drivers. *J Sleep Res* 1996;5:229–237.

23. Stoohs RA, Bingham LA, Itoi A, Guillerminault C, Dement WC. Sleep and sleep-disordered breathing in commercial long-haul truck drivers. *Chest* 1995;107:1275–1282.

24. Pack AI, Dinges DF, Maislin G. A study of prevalence of sleep apnea among commercial truck drivers. FMCSA Publication No. DOT-RT-02-030. Washington: FMCSA, 2002.

25. Shiomi T, Arita AT, Banno K, et al. Falling asleep while driving and automobile accidents among patients with obstructive sleep apnea-hypopnea syndrome. *Psychiatry Clin Neurosci* 2002;56:333–334.

26. Gurubhagavatula I, Maislin G, Pack AI. An algorithm to stratify sleep apnea risk in a sleep disorders clinic population. *Am J Respir Crit Care Med* 2001;164:1904–1909.

27. Maislin G, Pack A, Kribbs N, Smith P, Schwab R, Dinges D. A survey screen for prediction of apnea. *Sleep* 1995;18:158–166.

28. Flemons WW. Obsructive sleep apnea. *N Engl J Med* 2002;347:498–504.

29. Pack AI, Maislin G. Who should get treated for sleep apnea? *Ann Intern Med* 2001;134:1065–1067.

30. Piccirillo JF, Duntley S, Schotland H. Obstructive sleep apnea. *JAMA* 2000;284:1492–1494.

31. Lamphere J, Roehrs T, Witteg R, et al. Recovery of alertness after CPAP in apnea. *Chest* 1989;98(6):1364–1367.

32. Kribbs NB, Pack AI, Kline LR, et al. Effects of one night without nasal CPAP treatment on sleep and sleepiness in patients with obstructive sleep apnea. *Am Rev Respir Dis* 1993;147:1162–1168.

33. Aldrich M. Automobile accidents in patients with sleep disorders. *Sleep* 1989;12:487–494.

34. American Thoracic Society. Sleep apnea, sleepiness, and driving risk. *Am J Respir Crit Care Med* 1994;150:1463–1473.

35. Australasian Faculty of Occupational Medicine. *Medical Examinations of Commercial Vehicle Drivers.* Prepared for the National Road Transport Commission and the Federal Office of Road Safety, Sydney, Australia, 1997. *http://www.nrtc.gov.au/publications/ medstand.asp?lo=public.* Accessed Dec. 2, 2002.

6

Musculoskeletal Disorders

SAMUEL D. CAUGHRON, MD

There are few data on motor vehicle crash risk due to musculoskeletal disorders (MSDs), particularly among commercial motor vehicle operators. In the general driving population, data from a population-based 5-year retrospective study showed that the risk for at-fault motor vehicle crashes among drivers with licensing restrictions owing to MSDs was quite elevated (relative risk [RR] = 11.3, 95% confidence interval [CI], 2.39–53.3), as was that among drivers without restrictions (RR = 1.84, 95% CI = 1.14–2.98). The RRs for all motor vehicle crashes for those with MSDs but not restricted were elevated (RR = 1.59, 95% CI = 1.10–2.29), as were those for restricted drivers (RR = 4.51, 95% CI = 1.01–20.1) [1]. Thus, license restrictions may be appropriate to protect the public welfare. The examining physician should be aware of the nuances of the disease process(es) that may affect performance and the musculoskeletal work components of the job. Physical tasks may include lifting/carrying, prolonged sitting, twisting of neck and torso, squatting/crouching, and pushing/pulling. It is not the mandate of the commercial medical examiner to suggest treatment. This is best deferred to the driver's personal physician, since giving medical advice may establish a physician-patient relationship potentially fraught with medicolegal complications. In my experience, individuals with severe musculoskeletal problems seem to self-select themselves out of this profession, so I have rarely had to reject an applicant on these criteria.

Physical qualifications dictated by federal law (49 CFR 391.41) for commercial drivers state that a person shall not drive a motor vehicle unless he or she is physically qualified to do so [2]. The law has three references to musculoskeletal-related capabilities. In addition, there are medical advisory criteria for each standard that pertain to musculoskeletal problems. Subpart E, Section 391.41(b), specifically states:

A person is physically qualified to drive a motor vehicle if that person:

(1) Has no loss of a foot, leg, hand, or arm, or has been granted a skill performance evaluation certificate pursuant to Section 391.49;

(2) Has no impairment of:

(i) A hand or finger which interferes with pretension or power grasping;

or

(ii) An arm, foot, or leg which interferes with the ability to perform normal tasks associated with operating a motor vehicle;

or

(iii) Any other significant limb defect or limitation which interferes with the ability to perform normal tasks associated with operating a motor vehicle;

or

(iv) Has been granted a skill performance evaluation certificate pursuant to Section 391.49 and

then (3) Has no established medical history or clinical diagnosis of rheumatic, arthritic, orthopedic, muscular, neuro-muscular, or vascular disease which interferes with his ability to control and operate a motor vehicle safely.

The regulation describing the process for what had been formerly known as the limb waiver is 49 CFR 391.49. The process is now referred to as the skill performance evaluation certificate. The complete application process can be found at *http://www.fmcsa.dot.gov/safetyprogs/specert.htm.*

§ 391.49 Alternative physical qualification standards for the loss or impairment of limbs.

(a) A person who is not physically qualified to drive under Sec. 391.41(b)(1) or (b)(2) and who is otherwise qualified to drive a commercial motor vehicle, may drive a commercial motor vehicle, if the Division Administer, FMCSA, has granted a Skill Performance Evaluation (SPE) certificate to that person.

(b) SPE certificate.

(1) Application. A letter of application for an SPE certificate may be submitted jointly by the person (driver applicant) who seeks an SPE certificate and by the motor carrier that will employ the driver applicant, if the application is accepted.

(2) Application address. The application must be addressed to the applicable field service center, FMCSA, for the State in which the co-applicant motor carrier's principal place of business is located. The address of each, and the states serviced, are listed in Sec. 390.27 of this chapter.

(3) Exception. A letter of application for an SPE certificate may be submitted unilaterally by a driver applicant. The application must be addressed to the field service center, FMCSA, for the State in which the driver has legal residence. The driver applicant must comply with all the requirements of paragraph (c) of this section except those in (c)(1)(i) and (iii). The driver applicant shall respond to the requirements of paragraphs (c)(2)(i) to (v) of this section, if the information is known.

Musculoskeletal functions necessary to perform the job of a commercial driver include strength, agility, balance, coordination, and endurance. After long periods of relative physical inactivity while driving, a driver may be called upon to perform demanding physical tasks. Such tasks can involve lifting, pushing, or pulling to unload. Subsequently, the driver may be required to safely resume driving. Agility is required to view loads, mirrors, and equipment. Often, the drivers may need to be in difficult body positions to access connect-disconnect mechanisms, check wheels, or load. Even getting into a high truck requires balance and coordination. All of these tasks may be made more difficult by inclement weather. The very acts of driving, shifting gears, and operating the steering wheel require coordination and strength.

Risk factors for musculoskeletal occupational problems include lifting and forceful movements, awkward body posture, vibration, and non–work-related factors such as age, sex, psychological stresses, etc. These often exacerbate genetic or individual traits to increase the chance of discomfort during the act of driving [3]. The exact nature of the mechanisms involved, however, is often unclear. The National Institute for Occupational Safety and Health (NIOSH) is studying this area [4].

Proposed etiologies of injury include initial microtrauma, with callus formation altering the nutrient mechanisms, or tissue fatigue from continuous compression and stretching of the spinal structures [5].

Awkward body posture with rapid twisting can generate shear or rotational forces on the lower back, resulting in trauma. Prolonged sitting in poorly designed chairs with inadequate lumbar support or adjustability can result in intradiscal pressures significantly higher than compared with standing or the supine position [6]. An example of the stress on the driver is found in one study where the driver's body was flexed when lifting more than 60 percent of the time [7].

The truck driver's work requires sitting in a fixed posture for prolonged periods when driving. A total of 606 truck drivers belonging to a trade union were interviewed, and 63 subjects using the methods proposed by the Ergonomics of Posture and Movement Research Unit of the Clinica del Lavoro of Milan were examined. There was an elevated frequency of herniated disk, and the risk was four times higher compared with the control population. The frequency of functional spondyloarthropathy of the cervical and lumbar segments was particularly high, especially in the older age classes (71.4 and 35.7 percent, respectively) [8].

Whole-body vibration is recognized as having strong epidemiological evidence to be a risk factor for low back pain by NIOSH [4]. To date, there are no specific vibration standards or threshold limit regulations in the United States. A high prevalence of back pain, early degenerative changes of the spine, and herniated lumbar disc problems are consistently reported among drivers [3,9].

Non–work-related factors of age, gender, genetic, psychosocial, or anthropomorphic factors, etc., may be important. These are also potentially important in disability evaluations. These may influence the development of MSD in several ways [10]. They may increase muscle tension, influencing reporting or perception of discomfort. They may trigger a nervous system dysfunction because of underlying psychosomatic interaction or in some situations affect apparent causality, with impact on the severity, duration, and progression of the initial event.

Even treatment of MSDs, with both over-the-counter and prescription medications, can influence a driver's concentration and safety. Most acute injuries seem to be produced by lifting, pushing, and pulling. Musculoskeletal complaints appear in up to 54 percent of the population claiming disability [11], and truck drivers are noted to have almost twice the incidence of low back pain as the general population (22 percent) [12].

The medical examiner must keep all this in mind as he or she determines the length of time for which the medical certificate is given and whether a waiver or exemption may be necessary to allow a driver to drive commercially.

Those drivers with loss or impairment of a foot, leg, hand, or arm may be eligible for a Skill Performance Evaluation (SPE) certificate. The SPE certificate is granted by the Division Administrator of the Federal Motor Carrier Safety Administration (FMCSA), who makes the determination as to whether the driver, despite his or her impairment, is able to operate the commercial motor vehicle safely. If the medical examiner determines that a driver is otherwise qualified under Section 391.41(b)(3–13), he or she may indicate on the medical certificate that such a driver is medically qualified only if the medical certificate is accompanied by an SPE.

The advisory criteria for Section 391.41(b)(7) explain that "certain diseases are known to have acute episodes of transient muscle weakness, poor muscular coordination (ataxia), abnormal sensations (paresthesias), decreased muscular tone (hypotonia), visual disturbances, and pain, any of which may be suddenly incapacitating. The criteria go on to state that with such diseases, as the disease progresses, the episodes may become more frequent and more prolonged.

The more insidious diseases may cause atrophy, swelling, or weakness; therefore, the disability may not be acute but may be progressive to a point where the driver is unable to operate the vehicle.

An established history of a rheumatic, arthritic, orthopedic, muscular, neuromuscular, or vascular disease is present once a diagnosis of such a disease is made. Examiners must take into account four factors in determining a driver's medical qualification status:

1. The nature and severity of the individual's condition

2. The degree of limitation present

3. The likelihood of progressive limitation

4. The likelihood of sudden incapacitation

Only a driver whose current status is unlikely to interfere with the safe performance of a commercial driver's tasks should be certified. The examiner does have the option to qualify a driver for less than a 2-year period if he or she believes that, while currently safe to perform the job, progression of the disease may affect functional status during that time frame.

Potential Areas of Concern

Unlike many of the other medical conditions that may affect commercial driving, the FMCSA has not held a conference to address musculoskeletal diseases. Some of the neuromuscular diseases have been covered in the neurologic conference [13].

Rheumatic and musculoskeletal diseases include arthropathies, connective tissue disorders, back disorders, soft tissue rheumatism, bone disorders, sprains, and strains. They may be orthopedic, arthritic, muscular, neuromuscular, or vascular and may be of immune, infectious, traumatic, congenital, nutritional, hormonal, carcinogenic, degenerative, or unknown etiology. Musculoskeletal problems frequently occur concurrently with other medical problems and may be complicated by treatments and therapies [14].

Although a rheumatic or arthritic disease may be present, control with adequate medication and supportive care, however, usually will allow a commercial driver to work safely [15].

The commercial driver will have the same musculoskeletal conditions as the general public. Muscular disorders, including muscular dystrophy, multiple sclerosis, and acute injury, must be evaluated on an individual basis. The course of some neuromuscular diseases, such as multiple sclerosis, may be variable and require more frequent evaluations.

1. *Lacerations* are common, leaving telltale scars. Be sure to check for neurologic damage and decreased range of motion that may affect driving.

2. *Contusions and other soft injuries* may lead to compartment syndromes with decreased range of motion. If compartment syndrome is a concern, also evaluate peripheral pulses and neurologic function.

3. *Amputations* may be traumatic or due to complications of metabolic problems such as diabetes. Prosthetic devices and rehabilitation may provide the patient with excellent function, but these cannot replace the natural limb. Reimplantation may be seen primarily in upper extremity or hand injuries. The ability to perform job duties in such an individual must be evaluated, in many cases by functional testing.

4. *Entrapment syndromes* such as carpal tunnel syndrome involve the peripheral nerves and may cause resultant numbness,

paresthesias, pain, or loss of function; carpal tunnel syndrome is a common occupational problem. Repetitive-use injury is a controversial topic as to etiology and its relationship to specific tasks.

5. *Sprains and strains* of the ankle, wrist, elbow, shoulder, and knee may cause considerable functional impairment. If there is any question as to whether such an injury will interfere with safe work practices, it may be desirable to defer the qualification decision until the driver has reached maximal medical improvement.

6. *Tendonitis and bursitis* frequently increase with age. Gradual degeneration occurs, increasing the chance of acute irritation and pain with acute or nonspecific types. Placing stress on the tendons involved may indicate the severity of the symptomatic involvement.

7. *Rheumatic diseases*—The classification of rheumatic diseases is extensive, with more than 150 different diagnoses possible. Many of these diseases may cause pain, deformity, and limitation of motion. They may be exacerbated by physical trauma associated with vibration or by the combination of altered lifestyle, stress, and physical inactivity interspersed with overexertion associated with commercial driving. The musculoskeletal effects of each disease should be evaluated in terms of the job description provided by the employer or obtained from the examinee. The course and prognosis of the specific disease should influence the duration of the medical certificate. The physical evaluation in combination with the psychosocial evaluation should be used to arrive at a medical qualification decision. Histories may be inaccurate and diagnoses incomplete in some of these patients. Additional information from the driver's personal physician such as x-ray or laboratory reports are useful to consider in arriving at or supporting the qualifying decision.

Following is a brief review (in part) of some of the American Rheumatism Association's classification of rheumatic diseases [14]. Some issues of importance in examining the commercial drivers are also discussed.

   a. *Osteoarthritis* (degenerative joint disease) increases with age. Anatomic abnormalities, such as Heberden or Bouchard nodes, are not uniformly associated with clinical symptoms. The disease process commonly involves the fingers;

however, disease of the hips, neck, or knees can be disabling. Neurologic deficits may result from neck lesions.

b. *Traumatic arthritis* caused by injury to a joint, ligament, or meniscus may leave residual arthritis that is amenable to surgical intervention.

c. *Rheumatoid arthritis* can lead to severe deformity and disability. Some patients may go into remission, but most will proceed to further damage. Although the etiology is unknown, autoimmune or infectious factors may be present. Constitutional symptoms such as malaise, weakness, and fatigue also may occur. Peripheral swelling, joint pain, and limitation of motion are the most characteristic features of the illness. Associated diseases such as pericarditis or Sjögren's syndrome may occur. Subluxation of joints may occur, including cervical vertebrae, with subsequent pain and potential neurologic dysfunction. Flexion contractures, hyperextensibility, and boutonniere or swan-neck deformities, with loss of function, can occur. Look for accompanying entrapment syndromes. Rheumatoid arthritis is not always disabling.

d. *Psoriatic arthritis* can involve the spine. Consider this when a rash compatible with psoriasis is noted in a driver with arthritis.

e. *Spondyloarthropathies* represent a rare form of arthritis. Watch for stooped posture, which can affect the ability to see. Spondyloarthropathies also can affect the sacroiliac joints, with loss of lumbar lordosis. Nongranulomatous acute iritis may occur in 30 to 40 percent of patients. Aortitis and possible inflammatory lesions in the heart can lead to conduction disturbances. If there are clinical indications, consider obtaining an electrocardiogram. Neuropathy can be present secondary to spinal fractures or dural scarring.

f. *Reiter's syndrome* is seen in patients with a history of nonbacterial urethritis, inflammatory arthritis, and conjunctivitis. It can lead to progressive arthritis, with 20 to 30 percent limited motion.

g. *Gout and crystal arthropathies* may be acute and severe. They are generally monoarticular initially and may cause chronic trophic changes that are detectable on physical examination. Pseudogout presents with more variable symptoms of pain and swelling.

h. *Infectious arthritis* is rare and not usually a problem, except for residual arthritis, which may occur after treatment.

i. *Systemic connective tissue disorders* are a group of disorders caused by autoimmune problems.

   (1) *Systemic lupus erythematosus* may present with multiple symptoms, such as rash, arthritis, and polyserositis. Mental status changes, including acute psychosis, also may occur. Raynaud's phenomenon with vasospasm of the digits also may be seen.

   (2) *Scleroderma* is a multisystem disease characterized by fibrosis, which can cause tenosynovitis, Raynaud's phenomenon, decreased mobility, myalgia, and weakness.

   (3) *Polymyositis,* at times with skin lesions (dermatomyositis), presents predominately with weakness and may be abrupt in onset.

   (4) *Polymyalgia rheumatica and temporal arteritis* affect patients older than 50 years and are characterized by striking muscle aching and soreness.

8. *Back problems* are ubiquitous, affecting more than 90 percent of the population at some time. Facet syndromes and dural irritation, possibly aggravated by the increased spinal pressures found in the sitting position, may be noted [16,17]. Decreased range of motion may be found. Body habitus, posture, and physical conditioning all play a role in back pain [3].

   Range of motion determinations of the spine and a complete neurologic evaluation should be performed on any driver with a history of significant back injury or surgery. It may be desirable to obtain records from the treating physician to be certain that the driver is indeed released to work. Review of computed tomographic scans, magnetic, resonance images, functional capacity evaluations, or work-hardening reports may assist the examiner in this evaluation.

9. *Neck pain and cervical disk disease* are secondary only to backache in musculoskeletal afflictions. Range of motion must be evaluated because, as it decreases, it can affect a driver's ability to watch gauges, mirrors, and loads and, most important, the ability to see the road. In addition, evaluate upper extremity neurologic function. Disk protrusions may progress throughout

life. Initial minor problems occurring between ages 20 and 30 years can become more severe and progress to cervical nerve root syndromes as the individual ages [18].

10. *Congenital and other problems:*

   a. *Spina bifida* can be quite mild or can be related to a more severe neurologic deficit. Check for abnormal sensory findings or weakness. This is often a static problem.

   b. *Scoliosis,* or a curvature of the spine, due to vertebral abnormalities or asymmetrical fusion can lead to more frequent back pain when exacerbated by vibrational stress or respiratory compromise by deformity.

   c. *Metabolic disturbances* such as rickets, osteomalacia, scurvy, osteoporosis, hyperparathyroidism, or hyperpituitarism can result in weaker bones that are more prone to fracture. These diseases also may lead to limitation of motion if the individual is exposed to vibratory stress or vigorous activity.

   d. *Disuse osteoporosis* is detectable in 50 percent of all persons older than 65 years. Gross pathologic fractures are common, particularly in the cancellous long bones such as the neck of the femur, neck of humerus, distal end of the radius, and vertebral bodies. These changes also can result in chronic and acute back pain, which can be incapacitating.

   e. *Hyperpituitarism* may be suggested by large hands and mandible and increased frontal bossing.

   f. *Osteitis deformans* (Paget's disease) is a slowly progressive enlargement and deformity of multiple bones. It affects 3 percent of all persons older than 40 years. Severe bone pain can be present.

   g. *Granulomatous conditions* are rare and occur mainly in childhood. Collectively, they are referred to as skeletal reticulosis; these may be nonlipid or lipid disorders. This condition results in frequent fractures, and rarely does such a child reach adulthood.

11. *Neuromuscular disorders*—The participants in the Conference on Neurologic Disorders and Commercial Drivers believed that the current medical examination was insufficient for assessing neurologic disorders. They recommended that any driver with signs or symptoms of a neurologic disorder be referred to a neurologist for evaluation. Progressive neurologic diseases were

separated into two categories for disqualification (Table 6-1). Drivers with diseases in the first category are disqualified automatically, whereas those with neurologic disorders falling into the second category likely would be disqualified, but appeals were to be possible. This appeals process, however, was never implemented.

The appeals process described by the conference included an evaluation by a board-certified neurologist, neurosurgeon, or physiatrist. If a driver were to complete such an evaluation successfully, an on-the-road driving test would be required. Annual examination was recommended if such a driver was deemed medically qualified after the complete assessment. While these have not been implemented in law, the process is a possible guide to ensuring competence to drive if you have significant unanswered questions about the driver when you've completed your exam.

The Musculoskeletal History and Examination

The musculoskeletal examination of the commercial driver is an abbreviated examination. The focus is screening for elements that would restrict the driver or prevent safe driving. Since time is limited during this examination, the medical examiner must use information obtained

Table 6-1. Categories for neurologic disqualification*

Automatic Disqualification	Disqualification with Possible Appeal
Dementia	Multiple sclerosis
Motor neuron disease	Peripheral neuropathy
Malignant tumors of the central nervous system	Myopathy
Huntington's disease	Neuromuscular junction disorder
Wilson's disease	Benign brain tumor
	Dyskinesia
	Treatable dementia
	Cerebellar ataxia

*Categories recommended by the Conference on Neurologic Disorders and Commercial Drivers, August 1988.

from other resources or while observing the driver doing other tasks in the examiner's office.

Subjective data may include information from the patient or company, family, or accompanying friends who are willing to share information on the driver's status.

Objective data used to justify the examiner's conclusions come from

1. Observed behavior by you or your staff of the patient outside of your office, that is, coming into the office or returning to the parking lot. Some observations may include posture, limps, and signs of pain or lack of pain.

2. Observed behavior by you or your staff during accumulation of the history or other parts of the examination in your office.

3. Specifically targeted physical examination for the musculo-skeletal system done during your face-to-face examination of the patient.

Specific sites of attention are the neck, spine, arms, and legs. Testing for strength, range of motion, and neurologic status constitutes the basis of the examination. A methodical examination, either from the head down or from the toes up, helps to avoid errors of omission in conducting the examination.

The functional assessment of commercial drivers includes manual muscle testing for general strength, mobility and stability, ability to grip and turn a steering wheel, and evaluation of sensation. Simple tests of strength can be done in the office by asking the driver to imitate the motion pattern necessary to turn a 24-inch steering wheel, offering resistance throughout this pattern. Mobility is checked by giving resistance while the driver simulates patterns found at work (i.e., push, pull, twist at shoulder level, at each side, downward, bend, kneel, crawl, etc.). Some understanding of the driver's job description helps to guide the exam. Stability is tested by offering resistance to trunk, forward, backward, sides while driver is seated and instructed to maintain position. Shifting can be simulated with reciprocal movement of both lower legs, and right hand against resistance. If the driver steps up and down on a footstool several times you can evaluate climbing. Sensation exams for touch, position sense, and vibration especially in the feet and hands are useful.

A thorough review of testing procedures for abnormalities is beyond the scope of this book. The examiner should be familiar with common muscular syndromes and any of the components of a musculoskeletal

Table 6-2. Sample musculoskeletal evaluation for commercial drivers, by Samuel D. Caughron, MD*

1. Cervical spine: Observe alignment and symmetry. Palpate the neck, cervical spine, and paravertebral, trapezius, and sternocleidomastoid muscles. Strength is best determined against the opposing force of your hand. Evaluate range of motion:
   a. Chin to chest: 45°
   b. Chin to ceiling: 45°
   c. Ear to shoulder: 40°
   d. Chin to shoulder: 70°

2. Thoracic and lumbar spine: Observe for symmetry and the presence of normal cervical and lordotic curves. With the driver standing, palpate along the spine and paraspinal muscles. You may percuss the spine if you suspect tenderness. Ask the driver to bend forward and touch his or her toes. Observe for curves. Check for range of motion by:
   a. Flexion (bending forward to touch toes): 75 to 90°
   b. Hyperextension (back bend): 30°
   c. Bending to sides: 35°
   d. Rotation of upper trunk on waist: 30°

3. Shoulder: Inspect for symmetry and palpate the sternoclavicular and acromioclavicular processes, clavicle, scapulae, coracoid process, greater tubercle of the humerus, and biceps groove.
   Range of motion:
   a. Symmetrical shrug of shoulders (Note that cranial nerve XI is also evaluated with the shrugged shoulders.)
   b. Flexion (raising both arms forward and over the head): 180°
   c. Hyperextension (back bend): 40°
   d. Abduction (lifting both arms laterally and straight up over the head): 180°
   e. Adduction (swinging arm across front of body): 50°
   f. Internal rotation (both arms behind hips, elbows out): 90°
   g. External rotation (arms behind the head, elbows out): 90°

4. Elbows: Watch the carrying angle (usually 5–15°).
   Flexion is normal at 160° and extension at 180°.

examination as may be indicated. Combining the musculoskeletal examination with the neurologic examination allows you to best detect defects in function. A brief review of this author's view of the important elements of the musculoskeletal examination and examination criteria are in Table 6-2. More detailed information on the musculoskeletal examination can be found in other texts [19–22].

Table 6-2.   Sample musculoskeletal evaluation for commercial drivers, by Samuel D. Caughron, MD* (*continued*)

5. Hands. Pronation and supination of the hand is checked with the elbow flexed at 90° by rotating the hand from palm side down to palm side up; it is usually 90°. Inspect the hands for deformity. Palpate for muscle bulk and tenderness. Grip strength should be about 60 lb. Check the metacarpals for flexion (90°) and extension (30°) and the carpals for extension (70°) and flexion (90°) at the wrist. Ulnar deviation is 55°, and radial deviation is 20°.

6. Hips: I usually check this as part of the normal bending and movement of the driver.
   a. Flexion (with the knee extended): 90°
   b. Flexion (with the knee bent): 120°
   c. Normal extension: 30°
   d. Internal rotation (supine with the bent knee rotating inward): 40°
   e. External rotation (supine with one foot on the other leg and the knee turned outward): 45°

7. Legs and knees: Inspect the lower leg alignment. The femur and tibia are usually less than 15° out of alignment. Check for weakness of the quadriceps by applying opposing force to knee flexion.
   Bending the knee should reveal 130° of flexion.
   Expect 15° in hyperextension.

8. Feet and ankles: Observe the patient bearing weight. Observe the contour of the ankle and the position of toes. Watch for excessive pronation or inversion of the ankles. Check the Achilles tendon. Bend and straighten the toes. Check range of motion with the driver sitting.
   a. Foot dorsiflexion (pointing the foot toward the ceiling): 20°
   b. Foot plantar flexion (pointing the foot toward the floor): 45°
   c. Ankle inversion: 30°
   d. Ankle eversion : 20°
   e. Abduction: 10°
   f. Adduction (rotating the ankle): 20°

*The range of motion examples I've used are rough guidelines for the normal exam [19].

References

1. Diller E, Cook L, Leonard D, Reading J, Dean JM, Vernon D. *Evaluating Drivers Licensed With Medical Conditions in Utah, 1992–1996*. Technical Report No. DOT HS 809 023. Washington: National Highway Traffic Safety Administration, June 1999.

2. U.S. Department of Transportation, Federal Highway Administration. *Title 49 of the Code of Federal Regulations 391.41 and 391.49*. Washington: Office of Motor Carriers, 2002.

3. Johanning E. Evaluation and management of occupational low back disorders. *Am J Industrial Med* 2000;37:94–111.

4. National Institute for Occupational Safety and Health. Executive summary: Low back and musculoskeletal disorders; evidence for work-relatedness. In: Bernard BP, ed. *Musculoskeletal Disorders (MSDs) and Workplace Factors/TOC*. Cincinnati, Ohio: National Institute for Occupational Safety and Health, July 1997.

5. Frymoyer J. Back pain and sciatica. *N Engl J Med* 1988;318:291–300.

6. Marras WS, Lavender SA, Leurgans SE, et al. Biomechanical risk factors for occupational related low back disorders. *Ergonomics* 1995;38:377–410.

7. Van-der-Beek AJ, Frings-Dresen MH. Physical workload of lorry drivers: A comparison of four methods of transport. *Ergonomics* 1995;38(7):1508–1520.

8. Piazzi A, Bollino G, Mattioli S. Spinal pathology in self-employed truck drivers [in Italian]. *Med Lav* 1991;82(2):122–130.

9. Dupuis H, Zerlett G. Whole-body vibration and disorders of the spine. *Int Arch Occup Environ Health* 1987;59:323–336.

10. Bongers PM, de Winter CR, Kompier JAJ, Hildebrandt VH. Psychosocial factors at work and musculoskeletal disease. *Scand J Work Environ Health* 1993;19:279–312.

11. Chirikos T. *An Analysis of Compositional Trends in Social Security Disability Insurance Awards, 1960–1991*. New York: Cambridge University Press, 1993.

12. Guo HR, Tanaka S, Cameron LL, et al. Back pain among workers in the United States: National estimates and workers at high risk. *Am J Ind Med* 1995;28(5):591–602.

13. U.S. Department of Transportation, Federal Highway Administration. *Conference on Neurologic Disorders and Commercial Drivers*. Publication No. FHWA-MC-88-042. Washington: U.S. DOT, Federal Highway Administration, Office of Motor Carriers, 1988.

14. Kelly WN, Harris ED, Ruddy S, Sledge CB, eds. *Textbook of Rheumatology*, 6th ed. Philadelphia: WB Saunders, 2001.

15. Kilsey JL, Hardy RJ. Driving of motor vehicles as a risk factor for acute herniated lumbar intervetebral disks. *Am J Epidemiol* 1975;102:62–73.
16. Hansson TH, Keller TS, Spengler DM. Mechanical behavior of the human lumbar spine, II: Fatigue strength during dynamic compressive loading. *J Orthop Res* 1987;5:479–487.
17. Nachemson AL. Disc pressure measurements. *Spine* 1981;6(1):93–97.
18. Herington T, Morse L. *Occupational Injuries: Evaluation, Management, and Prevention.* St. Louis: Mosby, 1995.
19. Swartz M. Physical examination of the musculoskeletal system. In: *Textbook of Physical Diagnosis, History, and Examination,* 34th ed. Philadelphia: WB Saunders, 1997.
20. Palmer ML, Epler MI. *Fundamentals of Musculoskeletal Assessment Techniques.* Philadelphia: JB Lippincott, 1998:5–6.
21. Salter RB. *Textbook of Disorders and Injuries of the Musculoskeletal System,* 2nd ed. Baltimore: Williams & Wilkins, 1983.
22. Miller M, Kippel J, Dieppe P. *Review of Orthopaedics,* 2nd ed. Philadelphia: WB Saunders, 1996.

7

Neurologic Disorders

Kurt T. Hegmann, MD, MPH

Disorders affecting the nervous system and the capability for safe operation of commercial motor vehicles are quite common. Cerebrovascular disorders are the third leading cause of death in the United States [1]. Headaches, fatigue, vertigo, and dizziness are among the twenty most common reasons to visit a physician in the United States [2]. Together, these chief complaints comprise approximately 22,231,000 annual office visits (3.2 percent). Data suggest that some of these disorders present an increased risk for motor vehicle crashes [3]. Thus, the high prevalence of nervous system disorders combined with increased motor vehicle crash risk results in the need to frequently deal with such issues in the context of the commercial driver medical examination process.

Neurologic Disorders and the Commercial Driver Medical Examination Certification Process

Requirements

A commercial driver may not have an active seizure disorder. The driver must hear a forced whisper at not less than 5 ft. If audiometry is used, the better ear must not be more than 40 dB-A averaged at 500, 1000, and 2000 Hz. Hearing aids may be used to achieve these levels of hearing. The vision requirement is 20/40 or better in each eye, whether obtained by correction or not. However, there are many other disorders and problems that are recommended by the Conference on Neurologic Disorders and Commercial Drivers [4] as disqualifying due to diagnosis, prognosis, or complications of treatment.

Recommendations

Neurologic and psychiatric disorders were addressed in separate conference reports that were recommendations of committees of experts to the U.S. Department of Transportation for dealing with these problems [4]. The specific sets of recommendations were never implemented, yet they form the basis for handling these problems and approaching patients with various disorders.

Invariably, the first issue is to secure an accurate diagnosis [4]. Subsequently, it was recommended that three categories of risk be addressed:

1. The prognosis/risk of the disease itself

2. The risk of a complication or recurrence

3. The risk of a therapeutic complication

At any step during this proposed, sequenced evaluation, a commercial driver may be disqualified based on the information obtained at that step (Table 7-1). For example, a driver may have a diagnosis such as presumptive Alzheimer's disease, a condition recommended to be disqualifying by the conference report. In that case, the driver would not be allowed to drive. Conversely, a driver with a relatively benign disorder, such as a benign tremor not necessitating treatment, probably would be allowed to drive.

For relatively stable and benign conditions, such as a driver with a diagnosis of mild Parkinson's disease, easily managed by medication and without substantial potential for impairment while driving, an "appeals process" was proposed, though never implemented, that would allow the driver to retain certification.

Table 7-1. Commercial driver medical examination guidelines for neurologic disorders*

---

1. Diagnosis

2. Disability

3. Mental disability

4. Approved to drive

Note: Disqualification may occur at any step in the proposed process.
*Conference on Neurologic Disorders and Commercial Drivers [4].

This conceptual framework is still useful in evaluating the commercial driver. If one encounters drivers with some of these conditions, particularly in areas of uncertainty about driving risk, referrals to gain learned opinions are frequently helpful in this process.

Proposed Cognitive Screen Components

The Conference on Neurologic Disorders and Commercial Drivers [4] recommended a cognitive-impairment screen to assess an individual's ability to perform mental functions. The proposed screen includes evaluation of

1. Orientation to person, place, and time
2. Verbal and nonverbal intellect
3. Visual and verbal memory
4. Visuoperceptive abilities, including visual resolution, fields, and visuospatial performance
5. Language ability, including comprehension, ability to repeat, and reading ability

For the basic commercial driver medical examination, it was recommended that the physician

1. Note the comportment and level of alertness, comprehension of questions, and insightfulness of responses.
2. Have the applicant read a standard paragraph or sentence aloud and state what it means.
3. Have the applicant spontaneously write a sentence.
4. Have the applicant copy a standard complex geometric figure.
5. Administer a standard Mini-Mental Status Examination whenever there is doubt about the capabilities.
6. Test visual acuity with a Snellen chart.
7. Assess visual fields separately in each ocular quadrant by finger counting to confrontational fields.
8. Look for evidence of hemineglect of sensory stimuli by double simultaneous stimulation in the visual hemifields and in the tactile modality.

Doubtless, the commercial driver medical examination is not currently performed with all of the tests noted in this list. Still, several of these items are generally performed (*), and in those situations where further investigation is desired, the list may serve as a useful reminder of potential avenues for additional testing.

The task of writing is frequently assessed with the standard questionnaire. Particularly, all positive responses to the review of systems portion of the form should be further explained in the form's section following the checklist. One may consider observing the driver complete the form for those who failed to write additional, requisite information in this area of the form. A complete Mini-Mental Status Examination is also not generally performed because it would usually be of low yield in a setting outside of significant impairment, yet it may be of assistance in certain cases where questions particularly concerning global impairment arise. Should abnormalities be discovered or suspected through this process, then some or all of the items recommended by the conference report, as well as other clinical tests, may be needed.

The physical examination recommendations in the conference report are detailed, time-consuming, and likely of low yield for routine implementation. However, they too may be of assistance for use in those situations where additional investigation seems to be needed. The conference report recommendations include the following tests:

1. Cranial nerves (CNs)—visual fields, presence of hemianopia or central scotopia, denial of any field, diplopia, or oscillopsia; significant hearing deficits

2. Sensory nerves—pain, paresthesias, or dysesthesias because these can distract the driver's attention; any hypesthesia or anesthesia likely to impair fine-skilled use of the hands, arms, or legs; disturbances in proprioception

3. Motor nerves—strength, range of motion, reflexes, skill, dexterity, and reaction time; involuntary movements or alterations in tone (spasticity, rigidity); gait (normal and tandem)

The following list of screening tests for neurologic disorders is recommended for routine use by this author for commercial driver medical examinations (with additional tests performed as indicated):

1. Snellen, Ishihara, depth perception, and peripheral visual fields (CN II)

2. Pupillary appearance, reactivity to light, and constriction (CN II)

3. Extraoccular movements (CNs III, IV, and VI)

4. Facial expression and symmetry (CN VII)

5. Tympanic membranes and middle ear appearance (CN VIII)

6. Audiometry, or at least a forced whisper test (CN VIII)

7. Gag reflex (CN IX)

8. Palatal movement (CN X)

9. Tongue movement (CN XII)

10. Gait

11. Squat and standing strength, qualitative grip strength

12. Ranges of motion of the back (flexion), neck (all planes), shoulders, elbows, wrists, and phalanges; appearance of same

13. Deep tendon reflexes (patellar)

14. Romberg

15. Babinski

16. Speech

17. Comprehension, understanding, communication, and interaction

Disqualifying Conditions

Tables 7-2 through 7-5 list those conditions that were recommended to be automatically disqualifying in the Conference on Neurologic Disorders and Commercial Drivers. Although the lists are fairly lengthy, they are not exhaustive, since there are many rare conditions. These lists provide a basis for dealing with nearly all drivers, since persons with rare conditions most commonly would be categorized in a disease group (e.g., motor neuron diseases) and the recommendation could be inferred from the recommendations for similar conditions. It should be remembered, however, that none of these conditions, with the exception of active seizure disorder, is considered to be absolutely "disqualifying" by the Federal Motor Carrier Safety Administration (FMCSA); rather, these were the recommended actions for each of these disorders by the panel of experts.

Table 7-2. Automatically disqualifying neurologic disorders*

Legally incompetent	Construction apraxia
Major psychiatric disorder	Amnestic problems
Aphasia, alexia	Frontal-lobe disorders
Dementia	Chronic cluster headaches
Cranial neuralgia	Migraines with neurologic deficits
Diplopia, oscillopsia	Ménière's disease
Nonfunctioning labyrinth	Hemineglect, right to left disorientation
Labyrinthine fistula	Hemianopia/hemineglect of the visual field

*As recommended by the Conference on Neurologic Disorders and Commercial Drivers [4].

In Australia, syncope is considered to be incompatible with driving unless the cause is identified, treatment is successful, and compliance is confirmed [5]. In addition, narcolepsy is a disqualifying condition in Australia if the diagnosis is confirmed.

The Canadian Medical Association (CMA) [6] indicates that one syncopal episode that is explained and that is unlikely to recur may require no more than careful observation. Those with recurrent syncopal problems should not drive unless they have had successful treatment. Narcolepsy is believed to be incompatible with driving of commercial motor vehicles.

In Great Britain, individuals with syncope of unknown etiology may drive if 5 years have passed since the event and a specialist is in agreement with the decision to permit driving [7]. Individuals with narcolepsy are considered to have a completely disqualifying condition unless "a long period of control has been established," and then "licensing may be considered."

Cerebellar Degeneration

This group of disorders includes hereditary degenerative disorders, alcoholism, hypothyroidism, multiple sclerosis, infections, and consequences of tumors. Individuals with cerebellar ataxia were recommended to be disqualified from commercial vehicle operation by

Table 7-3.   Automatically disqualifying dementias*

Alzheimer's disease	Antihypertensive use
AIDS	Creutzfeldt-Jakob disease
Pick's disease	Syphilis
Parkinson's disease	Metabolic encephalopathy
Huntington's chorea	Alcoholism
Progressive supranuclear palsy	Depression
Cerebrovascular accident(s)	Granulomatous meningitis
Encephalitis	Vitamin B_{12} deficiency
Hypothyroidism	Heavy-metal toxicity
Organic-solvent toxicity	Tranquilizer use
Sedative use (prescribed and over-the-counter)	

Structural lesions

Tumor

Subdural hematoma

Multiple sclerosis

Stroke

Hydrocephalus

*These were recommended as disqualifying even if only "entertained" as a diagnosis for the presentatiosn of dementia.

the conference report. Generally, the same is true for the other disorders. However, it was believed that if the symptoms were mild or due to a treatable problem, then a second opinion from a neurologist was indicated.

Cerebrovascular Disease

Cerebrovascular disease is the third leading cause of death in the United States, although 87 percent of deaths occur in persons > 65 years of age [8]. There also is a high prevalence of people affected by these problems, with an estimate of more than 3 million stroke survivors [9]. An elevated risk of accidents in affected drivers has been reported [10]. Since some

Table 7-4. Automatically disqualifying neuromuscular diseases*

Motor neuron disease

Systemic peripheral neuropathy

Neuromuscular junction disease

Multiple dystrophy

Dermatomyositis

Metabolic muscle disease

Congenital myopathy

Myotonia

*As recommended by the Conference on Neurologic Disorders and Commercial Drivers [4].

problems occur at younger ages and the prevalence of these disorders is high, it is reasonable to infer that a commercial driver medical examiner will deal with this issue on a periodic basis.

Transient ischemic attacks (TIAs) are often one of the first manifestations of cerebrovascular disease, and the conference report recommended that a person with a history of TIAs be disqualified from driving a commercial vehicle interstate for 1 year because of the high rate of recurrence and/or stroke within the first year. Subsequent clearance by a neurologist was recommended.

Drivers with thromboembolic strokes involving the brainstem or cerebellum were recommended to be handled the same as those with

Table 7-5. Tumor and Parkinson's disease (proposed procedure)*

CNS tumors (primary or secondary)

1. Disqualify

2. Drivers with treated benign tumors may apply for an "appeal"

Parkinsonism

1. Disqualify

2. Drivers who are stable under treatment and compliant, with no on-off phenomena, no side effects, and no mental impairments, may "appeal"

*Conference on Neurologic Disorders and Commercial Drivers [4].

TIAs. However, strokes more commonly involve the middle/anterior cerebral distributions and have a worse prognosis. For such drivers, it was recommended that 5 years elapse prior to a neurology clearance examination to consider up to a 1-year certification, particularly if there is evidence of neurologic deficit. Drivers with deficits and stability such that a license can be granted should be recertified for no more than 1 year. Since most strokes involve areas such as the middle cerebral artery in those in their sixth or seventh decade, these are often career-ending events.

In Australia, drivers who have had a stroke are not believed to be qualified to continue driving a commercial vehicle [5]. A conditional license could be granted if the stroke was "caused by a condition which has now been satisfactorily treated. A satisfactory recovery from the stroke, including perceptual deficits, must also be demonstrated." Two or more TIAs preclude driving, but a conditional license may be granted if there is a 6-month TIA-free interval and the underlying cause has been "removed." For drivers with one TIA, referral to an approved specialist is required for certification.

In Canada, the CMA recommends that a driver not operate a vehicle for at least 1 month after a stroke [6]. They are not to drive if they have a TIA until a medical assessment is performed, even if there are no residua.

In Great Britain, the regulations recommend at least 12 months without driving a commercial vehicle after either a stroke or a TIA [7]. Licensure may be considered after that time if there is "full and complete recovery, and there are no other significant risk factors."

Dementias

Data on the motor vehicle crash risk for commercial drivers with dementia appear absent. This is not surprising as these individuals are mostly considered unqualified to drive. Relatively sparse data are available on crash risk for noncommercial drivers. Risks as high as 11-fold have been reported (odds ratio [OR] = 10.7, 95% confidence interval [CI] = 1.43–44.0) [11]. However, another study found mildly increased crash risk unless the disease was more advanced [12].

The conference report recommended that dementias be considered disqualifying conditions, even if the diagnosis has only been "entertained" (see Table 7-3). Thus, a patient who is being evaluated for the possibility of Parkinson's disease theoretically should be disqualified. The presence of tumors (benign or malignant), significant depression, and Alzheimer's disease all warrant disqualification. If the diagnosis is of a progressive disorder, the conference believed that there were "unequivocal grounds for disqualification." In such instances, computed tomography and magnetic resonance imaging (MRI) were considered "mandatory." For such drivers with mild symptoms or a slow rate of progression, as is often found in early Parkinson's disease, it was recommended that the examinee follow the "appeals process" (Table 7-6); the same appeals process was recommended for those with a treatable disorder, such as toxic dementia. If the neurologist and the examiner believe that the person can drive safely, then a shorter period of recertification, such as 6 months or 1 year, is recommended. As noted previously, however, this appeals process was never implemented. Nevertheless, the procedure for referring individuals with the potential to drive is logical and easily followed, except that education of the physician to whom the referral is made regarding driving requirements and regulations is often necessary.

Dementias are disqualifying conditions in Australia if the diagnosis or impairment is confirmed [5]. In Great Britain, the license must be revoked [7].

Extrapyramidal Disorders

These disorders are known to range in symptoms, severity, and prognoses. Common disorders include torsion dystonias (e.g., dystonia musculorum deformans, spasmodic torticollis, Meigs' syndrome, and blepharospasm), choreas (e.g., Huntington's, rheumatic fever, benign familial chorea, drug toxicities, or secondary to tumors and/or cerebrovascular accidents), myoclonus, tics, and benign essential (familial) tremor. Drivers with Wilson's disease or Huntington's chorea

---

Table 7-6. Appeals process for neurologic disorders*

---

1. Minor multiple sclerosis, mild dementia, some tumors, etc.

2. Magnetic resonance imaging

3. Neurology/physiatry examination

4. Simulated driving skills test

5. On-the-road driving test

Note: This process was proposed but never instituted. Disqualification could occur at any step in the process.

*Conference on Neurologic Disorders and Commercial Drivers [4].

are recommended to have "unequivocal grounds for disqualification." Other disorders require a careful assessment of the driver's status and a comparison between the person's capabilities and the demands of the job. Drivers with milder problems such as essential tremor, myoclonus, and focal dystonias were thought to be possible candidates for continued driving. However, annual recertification and neurologic or physiatric evaluations were thought to be required.

Headaches

Although headaches are common, only rarely are they thought to be a disqualifying condition (Table 7-7). A history of any of the following were believed to warrant a more detailed history: tension headache, migraine with or without neurologic deficit, cluster headache, posttraumatic head injury syndrome, drug-related headache, cranial neuralgia, atypical facial pain, cough headache, or exertional headache. Chronic cluster headaches, a rare condition, tend to bother an individual for an extended period of time (in contrast to more usual cluster headaches) and are considered disqualifying. However, if any headache is severe and incapacitating, or if medications are being taken that impair the ability to drive, then the headaches may be disqualifying. Migraines with neurologic deficits and cranial neuralgia also were classified as disqualifying conditions. Some data do exist to suggest higher accident rates among drivers with migraine headaches [13].

When evaluating an individual with headaches, it is recommended that the following information be elicited:

Table 7-7.   Headaches and vertigo*

Headaches

Chronic or incapacitating, *may* be disqualifying

Medication use may be problematic

Vertigo

Benign positional vertigo may requalify after 2 months

Acute/chronic vestibulopathy may requalify after 2 months

Ménière's disease and other chronic vertiginous problems are disqualifying

---

*As recommended by the Conference on Neurologic Disorders and Commercial Drivers [4].

1. Frequency and severity of the headache
2. Associated features
   a. Visual abnormalities: halos, scintillations, teichopsias, scotoma, quadrant anopsia, hemianopsia, diplopia, astereopsis, mosaic vision, visual distortion, or visual hallucinations
   b. Nausea and vomiting
   c. Dizziness, vertigo, dysequilibrium, and ataxia
   d. Mood swings from depression to agitation; transient psychosis
   e. Syncope
   f. Cognitive deficits: inattention, memory loss, confusion, disorientation, loss of concentration, speech disturbances, receptive deficits, or coma
   g. Motor deficits: ataxia, hemiparesis, hemiplegia, quadriparesis, or quadriplegia

The conference report recommended automatic disqualification for any of the associated features listed above. However, it seems that an individual who has a migraine once yearly, with nausea and vomiting, probably would be a reasonably good candidate for driving, provided there was reasonable warning prior to the emesis.

Special attention to the potential side effects from beta-blockers, antidepressants, and anticonvulsants used to treat headaches is also recommended.

Hearing Loss

Hearing acuity is obviously a less important sense than vision for the purposes of driving. Relatively few high-quality studies have been performed regarding the risks for motor vehicle accidents in hearing-impaired drivers, and almost none had been performed in commercial drivers. However, some studies do report an elevated risk for motor vehicle accidents in hearing-impaired drivers [14].

The required commercial driver medical examination screening for hearing acuity is the forced whisper test. In practice, a substantial number of examinations are accomplished with audiometry.

The basic regulatory criterion for hearing is the perception of a forced whisper at not less than 5 ft. Frequently, this is accomplished by asking the driver to repeat a series of random numbers. One of the problems with this test is that the typical examination room does not have 5 ft of distance from the patient's ear without either placing the patient in the corner of the room or requesting that the patient rotate his or her head position to test each ear. Although some firms request that their drivers be given a minimal screening, it is recommended that a formal request be made to the companies to screen with audiometry owing to the crude measure with the forced whisper combined with typically inadequately sized examination rooms. Thus, it is the opinion of this author that either audiometry or a handheld audioscope is preferable to the forced whisper test.

If a driver fails the forced whisper examination, then audiometry is recommended, and the requirement is that the individual have a corrected threshold of no worse than 40 dB-A averaged at 500, 1000, and 2000 Hz in the better ear. Thus, it is acceptable either to be deaf in one ear (provided that the other ear functions at the required threshold) or to achieve the required threshold through the use of hearing aids. Currently, these thresholds for hearing are not subject to interpretation or waivers. However, it should be noted that the previously stated intent of the FMCSA was to challenge the necessity of these functional levels with a waiver program. Such a program was never begun, however, because of lawsuits concerning the vision and diabetic waiver programs (see also "Visual Impairment" in this chapter and "Diabetes Mellitus Waivers" in Chapter 8).

In Australia, qualifications are somewhat more conservative, and disqualification occurs if the hearing threshold is greater than 40 dB-A in the better ear averaged at 500, 1000, 2000, and 3000 Hz [5]. Conditional licensure is granted for drivers who attain the hearing threshold requirements with hearing aids. The CMA recommendations are identical to those of the FHWA [6].

Multiple Sclerosis

Multiple sclerosis is one of the more common disorders encountered in the commercial driver certification process. The wide divergence in clinical course, treatment, impairment, cognitive involvement, and prognoses makes this disorder among the most challenging.

Data for the risk of motor vehicle crashes in commercial drivers are unavailable. Some data are available from the noncommercial driving population. A 10-year retrospective cohort study of 197 multiple sclerosis patients reported a relative risk (RR) of motor vehicle crashes requiring emergency department treatment of 3.4 (95% CI = 0.73–17.2); however, this failed to achieve statistical significance [15]. Some data based upon relatively small numbers of events suggest an elevated motor vehicle crash risk in those with multiple sclerosis who have concomitant cognitive deficits [16].

The conference report recommended that multiple sclerosis be considered a disqualifying condition. However, it was recognized that the severity of the problem, variability in the clinical presentation, and differing prognoses warranted the proposed "appeals" process for those with intermittent symptoms, mild deficits, and/or a stable clinical course. The conference report recommended an appeal under the following circumstances:

1. No signs of relapse or progression

2. No or only functionally insignificant neurologic signs and symptoms as determined by a neurologist

3. An MRI and triple-evoked potential studies are normal or do not reveal new lesions compared with prior evaluations made at least 1 year apart

4. No history of excessive fatigability or periodic fluctuations in motor performance, especially in relation to heat, physical and emotional stress, and infections

Since that conference report, the treatment of multiple sclerosis has evolved. Although far from curative, it is believed that some of the therapies have delayed disease progression. When in remission and early in the course of the disease, it may be that a driver can safely drive for some time without unnecessary risk to others. Significant judgment and the opinions of the treating neurologist are generally required in these circumstances.

In Australia, a conditional license may be granted if "the disability is limited to minor muscular weakness (subject to frequent re-assessment because of the progressive nature of such disorders)" [5]. The CMA recommends an evaluation of all drivers with disorders of coordination and muscle control to ascertain the degree of impairment [6]. For those "in the early stages of some of these conditions, no restriction on normal driving is necessary." In Great Britain, it is recommended that licensure not be granted if the disease is "progressive or disabling. If driving would not be impaired and [the] condition [is] stable, [drivers] may be licensed subject to annual review" [7]. This is the same guidance as for other chronic neurologic disorders.

Neuromuscular Diseases

Neuromuscular diseases are largely considered to be automatically disqualifying owing to interference with driving demands and poor prognoses. In the physical examination, particular attention should be paid to strength, sensory loss, and range of motion. Motor neuron diseases (e.g., spinal muscular atrophy, amyotrophic lateral sclerosis) should be disqualifying, as are systemic peripheral neuropathies (hereditary and acquired).

Myasthenia gravis is the main exception to automatic disqualification for the neuromuscular diseases. Although the conference report recommends that these neuromuscular junction diseases be considered disqualifying, most patients with myasthenia gravis, for example, likely can be completely managed. In such treated and stable individuals, recertification is generally justifiable.

Muscle diseases such as metabolic muscle diseases, muscular dystrophies, inflammatory myopathies (e.g., dermatomyositis, polymyositis, inclusion-body myositis), congenital myopathies, and diseases with abnormal muscle activity (e.g., myotonia, Isaac's syndrome, stiff-man syndrome) have disqualifying conditions. Confirmation of the diagnosis may be necessary; however, the conference report recommends that these be disqualifying conditions. It is recommended that any individual with a mild deficit from these types of diseases who is allowed to drive be given no more than a 1-year certification, and only after a careful evaluation.

In Australia, a conditional license may be granted if "the disability is limited to minor muscular weakness (subject to frequent re-assessment because of the progressive nature of such disorders)" [5]. The CMA recommends that these problems be handled in the same manner as multiple sclerosis [6]. In Great Britain, these disorders are handled in the same manner as Parkinson's disease or multiple sclerosis [7].

Parkinsonism

Motor vehicle crash data are not available for commercial drivers with Parkinson's disease. However, those with Parkinson's disease have been reported to have significant daytime somnolence (51 percent). The Epworth Sleepiness Scale helped somewhat to identify individuals falling asleep at the wheel (OR = 1.14, 95% CI = 1.06–1.24); however, an additional sleep scale (the "Inappropriate Sleep Composite Score") was more predictive (OR = 2.54, 95% CI = 1.76–3.66) [17]. This disorder typically occurs in older individuals, and thus concomitant diseases that may be disqualifying in and of themselves are possible and should be evaluated.

The conference report recommended that Parkinson's disease be disqualifying. Yet, presumably someone with mild, readily controlled Parkinson's symptoms and signs, no problems with dementia, no "on-off" phenomena, good compliance, and a lack of mental deficits may be considered for a shortened, time-limited certification.

In Australia, a conditional license may be granted if "the disability is limited to minor muscular weakness (subject to frequent re-assessment because of the progressive nature of such disorders)" [5]. The other possible scenario under which a conditional license may be granted is that the parkinsonism is drug induced and recovery is likely following cessation of treatment and that the "underlying cause for which the drugs were administered is not a cause for exclusion in its own right." The CMA recommends that these problems be handled in the same manner as multiple sclerosis [6]. In Great Britain, it is recommended that licensure not be granted if the disease is "progressive or disabling. If driving would not be impaired and [the] condition [is] stable, [drivers] may be licensed subject to annual review" [7]. This is the same guidance as for other chronic neurologic disorders.

Seizures

A history of epilepsy is one of the more common disorders (Table 7-8) encountered in the commercial driver certification process, as there is an approximately 3.0 percent cumulative incidence through age 74 years

---

Table 7-8.   Seizures and the commercial driver certification process*

Uncontrolled epilepsy is a disqualifier

Controlled epilepsy is a disqualifier

Remote history of seizures, on no medications, and seizure free for 10+ years: Recertify

History of one seizure, no recurrence, on no seizure medications for 5+ years: Recertify

History of febrile seizures as a child is *not* disqualifying

---

*As recommended by the Conference on Neurologic Disorders and Commercial Drivers [4].

for epilepsy, 4.1 percent for unprovoked seizure, and almost 10 percent for any convulsion disorder [18]. Although an active seizure disorder has been generally considered disqualifying for commercial drivers, the general driving population contains many individuals on antiepileptic medications. Thus, there are no data for safety in the commercial driving population, yet there are many data from the general driving population.

Data consistently demonstrate that drivers with an epileptic disorder have an elevated risk for motor vehicle crash, with typical estimates of approximately twice the risk of the general population for motor vehicle crashes [14,19–21]. A recent population-based study found similar estimates of risk; however, it found somewhat higher estimates for those involved in an at-fault accident whether on restrictions (RR = 2.39, 95% CI = 1.70–3.36) or not on restrictions (RR = 2.02, 95% CI = 1.08–2.27) [3]. By contrast, a 10-year Danish study found a sevenfold RR for motor vehicle crashes (RR = 7.0, 95% CI = 2.2–26.1) [22]. Severity of accidents has also been evaluated in a study evaluating emergency department treatment, with even stronger measures of risk (rate ratio = 7.01, 95% CI = 2.18–26.13), although the study was relatively small [22]. There also are data suggesting that those with epilepsy have experienced seizures while driving (33.3–39.2 percent) and report having experienced accidents while driving (17.3–26.7 percent) [23,24]. Seizure ablative therapy has not been found to be completely successful in those who also discontinue antiepileptic treatment, with reported 14 percent 2-year and 36 percent 5-year recurrence rates [25].

A history of childhood febrile seizures is the sole exception to concerns about a seizure history. A history of febrile seizures is considered nondisqualifying. All other histories of seizure disorders necessitate careful investigation of the condition. Controlled or uncontrolled epilepsy is considered to be a completely disqualifying condition. Although a history of any seizure disorder is a complete disqualifier, there are some exceptions.

When an individual has had only one seizure, has been off medications for 5 years, and has remained seizure free, that driver may be considered for qualification. Drivers with a seizure disorder history, off medications for 10 years, and remaining seizure free may be considered for qualification as well.

It may be noteworthy that there is evidence that most of the recurrence of seizures occurs within the first 2 years after cessation of antiepileptic agents [26], although the best data are in children and there are few data for adults [27]. Reported risk factors for recurrence include [28,29]:

- Partial seizures
- Myoclonic seizures
- Tonic-clonic seizures
- Young age at onset
- Experienced more seizures
- Longer treatment of seizures

- Seizure occurrence while on treatment
- Abnormal electroencephalogram
- Poor intellectual function
- Duration of treatment

In Australia, epilepsy precludes commercial vehicle driving; however, it is believed that a person could drive if he or she has been free of seizures for 5 years while off anticonvulsant medications [4]. It is also theoretically possible to grant a conditional license if the epilepsy is "so well controlled as to reduce the risk of a convulsion to that of any member of the general population," which seems to be virtually unattainable in nearly all cases. Single provoked seizures are also not believed to preclude commercial vehicle licensing. The CMA recommends against allowing epileptic drivers to operate commercial vehicles [6]. Those with a solitary seizure are believed to be able to be certified if seizure free for 1 year, and those with an epileptic history off medications and seizure free for 5 years are believed to be able to be certified. Those seizure free while on medications for 10 years are also believed to be able to drive commercial vehicles.

In Great Britain, the regulations require that drivers remain free of seizures for 10 years without anticonvulsants to be considered for certification [7]. For an unprovoked seizure, 10 years without an additional seizure is required to resume commercial driving. If the solitary seizure is due to alcohol use or medications, 5 years without an additional seizure is required.

Sleep Apnea

Sleep apnea is dealt with in the conference report on neurologic disorders as well as the conference report on pulmonary disorders. See Chapter 5 for a thorough discussion of this topic.

Transient Global Amnesia

Transient global amnesia is a condition believed to be due to cerebral ischemia that causes an episode of amnesia and confusion, with the patient recovering without sequelae. It is recommended that such a person be evaluated carefully with an electroencephalogram and psychiatric evaluation. If the evaluations are unremarkable, no restrictions are recommended, since the condition is then thought to be benign.

In Great Britain, driving should cease if there are two or more episodes [7]. After one episode, however, the driver is not required to surrender his or her license.

Traumatic Brain and Spinal Cord Injuries and Intracranial Bleeding

Problems related to traumatic brain injuries are generally due to lingering deficits (e.g., paresis or seizures) rather than the diagnosis, as they tend not to be progressive conditions. If there is no deficit, no special evaluations or time limits are recommended. However, the examiner may institute a different time frame for recertification if he or she believes that this is indicated. The conference report recommended that the evaluation be performed by a neurologist and include a physical examination, neurologic examination, neuro-ophthalmologic evaluation, and neuropsychological testing. If there is a deficit, annual follow-up evaluations are recommended. Spinal cord injuries resulting in paraplegia should result in disqualification. If weakness is present following a spinal cord injury, an assessment should be made to determine whether there is an impairment that would interfere with the safe operation of a motor vehicle. It is believed that the presence of a deficit should allow for no more than a 1-year certification, if at all.

In Australia, someone with more than 24 hours of altered consciousness or a serious head injury is not qualified to drive a commercial vehicle until assessed [5]. The assessment may include medical examination, neuropsychological testing, and/or a practical driving test. The CMA believes that minor injuries would not impair driving capability for more than a few hours [6]. It recommends that drivers with a more serious injury "should always be fully evaluated before driving is resumed."

In Great Britain, a specialist evaluation is recommended to assess such drivers [7]. The two primary complications to be addressed are epilepsy risk and driver performance. The threshold for epilepsy risk is a 2 percent risk estimate. For extradural intracranial hematomas without cerebral damage, 1 year without commercial vehicle operation is recommended. For individuals with cerebral damage or intracerebral bleeding, license revocation is recommended, and reinstatement depends on a specialist examination focusing particularly on the epilepsy risk threshold. Chronic subdural hematomas require 6 months to 1 year off depending on clinical features. Subarachnoid hemorrhage requires 6 months off and reinstatement only if an angiography is normal and the driver remains symptom free. If a craniotomy is required for a cerebral aneurysm, then 1 year without driving is recommended if the recovery is complete; revocation is recommended if recovery is incomplete. If the aneurysm is in the middle cerebral artery distribution, however, then 18 to 24 months away from driving is required for those without a residual deficit. For those with an incidental intracranial aneurysm, it is recommended that the license be revoked. However, if a specialist assessment assures a low risk for hemorrhage, then driving may resume. If an intracranial arteriovenous malformation (AVM) is diagnosed, the license is recommended to be revoked. If the epilepsy risk is believed to be less than 2 percent and the AVM is thought to be treated successfully, then such individuals are believed to be capable of driving with the approval of a specialist.

Tumors

Treated, benign central nervous system (CNS) tumors generally provide no long-term certification limitations provided there is no neurologic deficit or seizure disorder.

However, malignant CNS tumors do present significant problems that generally necessitate disqualification. Individuals with metastases should be considered disqualified permanently because they are unlikely to have a good prognostic outcome. Occasionally, individuals with malignant primary CNS tumors may be recertified after adequate treatment, complete cure, and no untoward effects (e.g., seizures, paresis, coordination abnormalities). A waiting period of several years prior to recertification, however, seems wise. Clearance by a neurologist is recommended.

The CMA recommends that benign tumors that have been treated and without deficits do not usually require prohibition from driving [6]. If a seizure occurs in the process of treatment, then a 1-year seizure-free period is required. An individual assessment is believed to be needed after treatment for a malignant tumor.

In Great Britain, the license is to be surrendered, and a driver may be considered for reinstatement 10 years after surgery with successful removal or cure of histologically benign tumors [7]. Drivers with gliomas are recommended to be permanently disqualified. Those with histologically malignant tumors (e.g., medulloblastoma) are recommended to be disqualified for at least 5 years. If the problem is an acoustic neuroma or meningioma, then driving may be resumed provided there are no disabling symptoms. A 6-month disqualification from driving after craniotomy for pituitary tumors is recommended, provided there are no visual field defects.

Vertigo

Acute labyrinthitis is likely the most common type of vertigo. As it is an acute and self-limited disorder, it is unlikely to result in long-term impairment or crash risk. The conference report recommends disqualification for 2 months; however, some individuals are symptom free within a week.

Drivers with acute and chronic vestibulopathies are recommended for recertification after being symptom free for 2 months. Individuals with chronic progressive vestibular diseases or permanent dysfunction, such as Ménière's disease, labyrinthine fistulas, and nonfunctioning labyrinths, are considered to have completely disabling conditions. (In contrast, the CMA does not recommend withdrawing a commercial license for individuals with chronic progressive vestibulopathies [6].)

The conference report recommended evaluation by a neurologist and careful assessment of drivers having these disorders. However, it seems that an individual with a clear case of acute labyrinthitis and complete resolution of symptoms would be a good candidate for recertification by the commercial driver examiner without universal neurologic clearance. Nevertheless, a time-limited certification for 2 to 6 months may be indicated for the first certification period.

In Australia, a 30-second Romberg test is used to screen for vertigo, and anyone with a positive test is to be referred to an approved specialist rather than certified [5]. Drivers with recurrent vertigo of any cause are not certifiable for commercial vehicle operation. If free of attacks for 12 months, they can be reassessed. These criteria also seem to preclude those with acute labyrinthitis from driving for 12 months. The CMA advises that those with acute labyrinthitis not drive "until the condition has subsided or responded to treatment" [6]. Those with recurrent vertiginous problems "should not drive any class of motor vehicle until their symptoms have been controlled." Great Britain has taken a similar approach that requires that the condition be stable and symptom free for 1 year prior to consideration of licensure [7].

Visual Impairment

Monocular commercial drivers have reported motor vehicle crash rates that compare favorably with those of the general population or commercial vehicle drivers [30].

However, a population-based study of motor vehicle drivers found elevated crash risks whether the driver was unrestricted (RR = 1.27, 95% CI = 1.04–1.55) or restricted (RR = 1.35, 95% CI = 1.25–1.46). At-fault accident risks were further elevated whether unrestricted (RR = 1.52, 95% CI = 1.38–1.68) or restricted (RR = 1.56, 95% CI = 1.25–1.94) [3]. Elderly drivers with cataracts seem to have problems driving [31]. A small controlled study of diplopia generally failed to find significant differences in response and recognition times [32].

The commercial driver medical examination screens for vision with three screens: (1) the Snellen chart, (2) a color screen, and (3) a peripheral vision screen. The basic criterion to drive is that a driver have visual acuity of 20/40 or better in *both* eyes, whether corrected or not (i.e., if drivers can achieve 20/40 or better in only one eye, they do *not* meet the standard qualification, although a vision exemption may be possible; see Chapter 3). The applicant must be able to discern the colors red, amber, and green. Last, peripheral vision must be at least 70 degrees laterally in each eye. The capability to distinguish the three colors may not be waived, although owing to this fairly simple requirement, drivers with many types of color blindness are still able to drive commercial motor vehicles. The minimum requirement of 20/40 visual acuity in each eye also may not be waived. However, a detailed exemption application process has been instituted (see Chapter 3) for those who have at least 20/40 corrected visual acuity in the better eye.

A provisional waiver program for monocular drivers was begun in 1992 [33]. A total of 2686 drivers were enrolled in the waiver program prior to a court injunction that stopped further enrollments in the mid-1990s. Nevertheless, these drivers were allowed to continue to operate commercial motor vehicles but were followed as part of an uncontrolled study. To be eligible for enrollment in the original program, drivers were required to have operated a commercial vehicle safely for 3 years prior to enrollment, to have no licensure suspensions/restrictions, and to have a doctor's approval that they could operate such a vehicle safely. (For more details of the waiver programs, see "Diabetes Mellitus Waivers" in Chapter 8.) Drivers were then monitored for accident rates, fatality rates, and property damage estimates.

There were 2234 drivers participating as of November 1995, a total dropout rate of approximately 16.8 percent [33]. All measures of accident rates were lower for the waived drivers compared with the national accident rate. The total accident rate was 1.706 per million vehicle miles traveled (VMTs) compared with the national rate of 2.605 per million VMTs. The property damage accident rate was 1.284 versus 2.048 per million VMTs. The accident rate with injury(ies) was 0.408 versus 0.534 per million VMTs. The fatal accident rate was 0.013 versus 0.026 million

VMTs for the national rate. All achieved statistical significance, but these were calculated at 90 percent CIs.

Based in part on the preceding findings, drivers who were in the program after its termination were permitted to continue operating in interstate commerce provided the following conditions are met:

1. They receive an annual ophthalmologic/optometric examination.

2. The vision in the better eye is documented to be 20/40 or better.

3. Annual certification by a medical examiner indicates that the driver is otherwise physically qualified to drive a commercial vehicle for interstate commerce.

4. The driver provides a copy of the ophthalmologic/optometric evaluation to the medical examiner at the time of examination.

5. The driver provides a copy of the annual medical certification to his or her employer or retains it in his or her driver qualification file if self-employed.

Vision exemptions are now being considered provided the individual is able to demonstrate to the FHWA that the degree of safety is at least equal to that which would be present were the exemption not needed. (See Chapter 1 for discussion of the application process. Contact the FMCSA at 202-366-2990 for more information.

Monocular drivers may be conditionally certified in Australia [5]. The visual requirement is that the corrected visual acuity be at least 6/9 in the better eye. Conditional licenses also may be granted for those with partial visual field defects if the loss does not result in less than a 140 horizontal visual field. Individuals with a red perception difficulty (protan) are not qualified to drive. Diplopia is also disqualifying unless it is only present on extreme lateral gaze, in which case a conditional license may be granted.

Canadian requirements are at least 20/40 with both eyes opened and examined together and not less than 20/200 in the worse eye [6]. Visual fields of 120 degrees in the horizontal plane are required. There is no color standard requirement.

Requirements in Great Britain are that a driver must have corrected visual acuity of at least 6/9 in the better eye and 6/12 in the worse eye [7]. Additionally, the uncorrected acuity must be at least 3/60 in both eyes. Monocular drivers may not be certified by law, although there is a grandfathering provision for previously licensed drivers. It is recommended that permanent disqualification be rendered if there is diplopia, night blindness, or blepharospasm. The field of vision must be at least 120. Color blindness is not disqualifying.

Two aspects of licensure for monocular drivers deserve further mention. The first is that a careful scrutiny of symptoms and problems with the remaining functional eye must be undertaken as part of the commercial driver medical examination. The second is that reliance on the neck range of motion to achieve a functional visual field is underrecognized. It is recommended that assessment of monocular drivers include an assessment of functional visual field by including a focused examination of the neck for axial rotation range of motion in the direction of the compromised eye.

References

1. National Center for Health Statistics. *Health, United States, 1994.* Publication No. DHHS (PHS) 95-1232. Hyattsville, MD: U.S. Public Health Service, 1995.
2. Schappert SM. National Ambulatory Medical Care Survey: 1989 summary. *Vital Health Stat 13* 1992;110:1–80.
3. Diller E, Cook L, Leonard D, Reading J, Dean JM, Vernon D. *Evaluating Drivers Licensed with Medical Conditions in Utah, 1992–1996.* Technical Report DOT HS 809 023. Washington: National Highway Traffic Safety Administration, June 1999.
4. U.S. Department of Transportation, Federal Highway Administration. *Conference on Neurologic Disorders and Commercial Drivers.* Publication No. FHWA-MC-88-042. Washington: U.S. DOT, Federal Highway Administration, Office of Motor Carriers, 1988.
5. Australasian Faculty of Occupational Medicine. *Medical Examinations of Commercial Vehicle Drivers.* Prepared for the National Road Transport Commission and the Federal Office of Road Safety, Sydney, Australia, 1997. *http://www.nrtc.gov.au/publications/assessment.pdf.* Accessed Dec. 9, 2002.
6. Canadian Medical Association. *Physicians' Guide to Driver Examination.* Ottawa, Canada. *http://www.cma.ca/cma/common/displayPage.do?pageId=/staticContent/HTML/publications/catalog/driversguide/index.htm.* Accessed Dec. 9, 2002.
7. Driver and Vehicle Licensing Agency. *At-a-Glance Guide to the Current Medical Standards of Fitness to Drive.* Swansea, England: Drivers Medical Unit, DVLA. *http://www.dvla.gov.uk/at_a_glance/content.htm* accessed Dec. 9, 2002.
8. U.S. Preventive Services Task Force. *Guide to Clinical Preventive Services,* 2nd ed. Baltimore: Williams & Wilkins, 1996.

9. Gresham GE, Duncan PW, Stason WB, et al. *Post-Stroke Rehabilitation.* Clinical Practice Guideline No. 16 (AHCPR Pub. No. 95-0662). Rockville, MD: Agency for Health Care Policy and Research, 1995.

10. Hansotia P. Seizure disorders, diabetes mellitus and cerebrovascular disease: Considerations for older drivers. *Clin Geriatr Med* 1993;9(2):323–339.

11. Zuin D, Ortiz H, Boromei D, Lopez OL. Motor vehicle crashes and abnormal driving behaviors in patients with dementia in Mendoza, Argentina. *Eur J Neurol* 2002;9:29–34.

12. Dubinsky RM, Stein AC, Lyons K. Practice parameter: Risk of driving and Alzheimer's disease (an evidence-based review): report of the Quality Standards Subcommittee of the American Academy of Neurology. *Neurology* 2000;54:2205–2211.

13. Lerman Y, Matar M, Lavie B, Danon YL. Effect of valvular heart diseases, migraine headaches, and perianal diseases on the risk of involvement in motor vehicle crashes. *J Trauma* 1995;39(6):1058–1062.

14. Songer TJ, LaPorte RE, Palmer CV, et al. *Hearing Disorders and Commercial Motor Vehicle Drivers.* Report No. FHWA-MC-93-004. Washington: U.S. DOT, Federal Highway Administration, Office of Motor Carriers, 1992.

15. Lings S. Driving accident frequency increased in patients with multiple sclerosis. *Acta Neurol Scand* 2002;105:169–173.

16. Schultheis MT, Garay E, Millis S, DeLuca J. Motor vehicle crashes and violations among drivers with multiple sclerosis. *Arch Phys Med Rehabil* 2002;83:1175–1178.

17. Hobson DE, Lang AE, Martin WRW, Rasmy A, Rivest J, Fleming J. Excessive daytime sleepiness and sudden-onset sleep in Parkinson disease. *JAMA* 2002;287:455–463.

18. Hauser WA, Annegers JF, Rocca WA. Descriptive epidemiology of epilepsy: Contributions of population-based studies from Rochester, Minnesota. *Mayo Clin Proc* 1996;71:576–586.

19. Hansotia P, Broste S. The effects of epilepsy and diabetes mellitus on the risk of automobile accidents. *N Engl J Med* 1991;324:22–26.

20. Hornio A. Does epilepsy mean higher susceptibility to traffic accidents? *Acta Psychiatr Scand* 1961;150(suppl):210–212.

21. Krumholz A, Fisher RS, Lesser RP, Hauser WA. Driving and epilepsy: A review and reappraisal. *JAMA* 1991;265(5):622–626.

22. Lings S. Increased driving accident frequency in Danish patients with epilepsy. *Neurology* 2001;57:435–439.

23. Berg AT, Vickery BG, Sperling MR, et al. Driving in adults with refractory localization-related epilepsy. *Neurology* 2000;54:625–630.

24. Gastaut H, Zifkin BG. The risk of automobile accidents with seizures occurring while driving: Relation to seizure type. *Neurology* 1987;37:1613–1616.

25. Schiller Y, Cascino GC, So EL, Marsh WR. Discontinuation of antiepileptic drugs after successful epilepsy surgery. *Neurology* 2000;54:346.

26. Emerson R, D'Souza BJ, Vining EP, Holden KR, Mellits ED, Freeman JM. Stopping medication in children with epilepsy: Predictors of outcome. *N Engl J Med* 1981;304:1125–1129.

27. Sirven JI, Sperling M, Wingerchuk DM. Early versus late antiepileptic drug withdrawal for people with epilepsy in remission (Cochrane Review). In: *The Cochrane Library.* Issue 4 2001. Oxford.

28. Medical Research Council Antiepileptic Drug Withdrawal Study Group. Randomized study of antiepileptic drug withdrawal in patients in remission. *Lancet* 1991;337(8751):1175–1180.

29. Medical Research Council Antiepileptic Drug Withdrawal Study Group. Prognostic index for recurrence of seizures after remission of epilepsy. *BMJ* 1993;306(6889):1374–1378.

30. Decina LE, Breton ME, Staplin L. *Visual Disorders and Commercial Drivers.* Publication No. FHWA-MC-92-003. Washington: U.S. DOT, Federal Highway Administration, 1991.

31. Owsley C, Stalvey BT, Wells J, Sloane ME, McGwin G Jr. Visual risk factors for crash involvement in older drivers with cataract. *Arch Ophthalmol* 2001;119(6):881–887.

32. White JF, Marshall SC, Diedrich-Closson KL, Burton AL. Evaluation of motor vehicle driving performance in patients with chronic diplopia. *J AAPOS* 2001;5:184–188.

33. Office of Motor Carrier Research and Standards. *Qualification of Drivers: Vision and Diabetes.* Technical Brief. Publication No. FHWA-MCRT-99-017. Washington: U.S. DOT, Federal Highway Administration, September 1999.

Additional References

Laux LF, Brelsford J. *Age-Related Changes in Sensory, Cognitive, Psychomotor and Physical Functioning and Driving Performance in Drivers Aged 40 to 92.* Washington: AAA Foundation for Traffic Safety, 1990:1–58.

Rehm CG, Ross SE. Syncope as etiology of road crashes involving elderly drivers. *Am Surg* 1995;61(11):1006–1008.

8

Endocrine Disorders

Kurt T. Hegmann, MD, MPH

Diabetes mellitus is one of the two most common disorders encountered in the commercial driver certification process (along with hypertension). Although the prevalence among commercial drivers is unclear, robust population-based estimates are available. The prevalence among those aged 40 to 74 years is 12 to 14 percent and among males aged 60 to 74 years is approximately 20 percent [1–4]. Worrisomely, approximately 50 percent of those were undiagnosed and were detected on blood testing.

Increasing attention is being devoted to a problem closely related to diabetes, the "metabolic syndrome" (also known as dysmetabolic syndrome X), owing to accompanying cardiovascular morbidity and mortality. See Table 8-1 for diagnostic criteria. Although probably not yet an issue that is under significant scrutiny in the process of most commercial driver certifications, it is one that likely warrants some awareness on the part of examiners.

Diabetes Mellitus and the Commercial Driver Medical Certification Process

Requirements

Interstate commercial drivers are currently prohibited from using insulin, although it may be approved for certain, select drivers in the future (see below). Other medical management of diabetes mellitus does not necessitate disqualification; however, a driver has to be under adequate control to be certified. Other complicating conditions may necessitate disqualification. All drivers must submit to urinalysis, although the thresholds for glucosuria demonstrate significant interindividual variation.

Table 8-1. Metabolic syndrome diagnostic criteria (*ICD-9-CM* 277.7)

Major criteria

- Acanthosis nigricans
- Waist circumference > 102 cm for men and > 88 cm for women
- Dyslipidemia (high-density lipoprotein cholesterol < 35 mg/dL for men and < 45 mg/dL for women, or triglycerides > 150 mg/dL)
- Hypertension
- Impaired fasting glucose or type 2 diabetes mellitus
- Hyperuricemia

Minor criteria

- Hypercoagulability
- Polycystic ovary syndrome
- Vascular endothelial dysfunction
- Microalbuminuria
- Coronary heart disease

Source: American Association of Clinical Endocrinologists.

Recommendations

It is recommended that applicants be asked questions about whether they have or had diabetes mellitus or "sugar problems." Any positive responses should result in many additional questions, including duration, medication(s), glycosylated hemoglobin results, diabetic education, end-organ complication(s), and frequency of physician examinations. From these questions, the examiner may then draw conclusions regarding the intensity of diabetic control and the risks for severe hypoglycemic reactions and better ascertain whether the individual is able to drive safely. Because of the great variability in the threshold for glucosuria, any nondiabetic individual who has glucose in the urine on dipstick urinalysis should necessitate further evaluation and at most should have a very short time-limited certification while undergoing further evaluation to ascertain whether the serum glucose level and/or glycohemoglobin is/are within the normal range, since the individual may well be completely out of control at the time of the screening test. Individuals found to be at the upper ranges of oral medication doses and in typically obese states of health should be cautioned that they may be nearing an early retirement because they may need to take insulin. This warning sometimes serves as a useful method for modifying poor eating and exercise habits among receptive individuals. Individuals who are thought to be in fair control probably should be certified for shorter time increments, e.g., 6 to 9 months, to allow for better surveillance of the situation and to encourage better control and compliance. While a change to yearly Federal Motor Carrier Safety Administration (FMCSA) examinations based on the diagnosis of diabetes mellitus is not mandatory, it would seem prudent to do so, particularly those with multiple risk factors for end-organ dysfunction.

Licensure Differences Between Jurisdictions

Diabetic drivers are handled significantly differently between various jurisdictions. Of 23 countries surveyed, 10 (43.5 percent), including Canada, Mexico, and the United States, prohibit insulin use in commercial motor vehicle drivers [5], although Canada has subsequently altered that policy. While the U.S. has been loosening the restrictions on diabetic commercial drivers and is considering allowing insulin use among some interstate drivers [6], Great Britain has been simultaneously tightening the requirements. It has been remarked that this highlights the lack of objective data upon which to found evidenced-based policies regarding diabetes mellitus [7]. Currently, drivers who use insulin are prohibited from commercial vehicle licensing in Great Britain, with "grandfathering" of some insulin-using drivers who were licensed prior to January 4, 1991 [8]. Great Britain also requires satisfactory control, recognition of warning symptoms, and a lack of end-organ problems that would preclude safe driving.

The Canadian Medical Association recommends annual examinations for diabetics [9]. For those without insulin for treatment, they are to have a good understanding of the diseases, comply with treatment, and remain under "regular medical supervision." Those on insulin "can have great difficulty maintaining the essential balance between insulin dose, food intake, and physical exertion" due to irregular work, activity, and food. A few carefully screened insulin-using diabetics may be allowed to hold a commercial vehicle license only after a favorable consultation with a diabetologist. Detailed guidelines are in place, including medical records review (prior 24 months), evidence of diabetes education program attendance, physical examination (including ophthalmology/optometry), glycosylated hemoglobin levels within the prior 3 months, and 6 months of twice-daily glucose log results. Exclusions include no severe hypoglycemia in the prior 6 months, no hypoglycemia unawareness, no instability in the insulin treatment regimen (unable to drive for 1 month), no visual impairment, no progressive proliferative retinopathy, no "obvious peripheral neuropathy with loss of function," no cardiovascular disease with dysrhythmias, and angina or myocardial infarction (prior year). Annual exams contain similar requirements, including two glycosylated hemoglobin measurements at 3-month intervals and 6 months of glucose logs. Drivers are not to drive if the glucose level falls below 108 mg/dL (6 mmol/L), and it is to be measured 1 hour prior to driving and every 4 hours while driving.

Australia prohibits diabetics from being certified as commercial vehicle drivers if they have hypoglycemic episodes, poor control, or target end-organ damage; insulin-using diabetics without end-organ damage or hypoglycemic episodes are considered certifiable in Australia by an approved specialist [10].

Many of the U.S. states permit some drivers to operate commercial vehicles [11] (Table 8-2). While some require additional monitoring if dietary management is initiated and some allow insulin use for intrastate commercial vehicle operation, others prohibit use of insulin. Familiarity with local regulations is essential.

Table 8-2. License status when an existing CMV driver develops diabetes

Treatment for diabetes	Lose license	Restrictions/ medical exam	No change	Don't know or no response
Begin insulin	9 (18%)	26 (52%)	14 (28%)	1 (2%)
Begin oral hypoglycemic	0 (0%)	22 (44%)	25 (50%)	3 (6%)
Begin dietary management	0 (0%)	14 (28%)	35 (70%)	1 (2%)

Source: U.S. Department of Transportation, Federal Highway Administration. Effect of limitation of various treatment protocols for diabetes mellitus on instrastate licenses in the 50 states. Washington, DC: Office of Motor Carriers. Publication No. FHWA-MC-92-012, 1992.

Screening for Diabetes Mellitus

Diabetes mellitus is one of most important disorders in the commercial driver certification process owing to prevalence [3,4], complications, and hazard potential to the public. With the sharply increasing prevalence of obesity, the prevalence of diabetes is expected to further increase. Currently, while the U.S. Preventive Services Task Force does not recommend screening individuals for diabetes mellitus [12], the American Diabetes Association recommends that screening be performed (Tables 8-3 and 8-4). Population-based screening studies have shown elevated risks for retinopathy starting at and rising sharply from fasting glucose levels of approximately 110 to 120 mg/dL [1]. Owing to significant evidence for efficacy of intensive glycemic control to prevent complications [13,14], further impetus to screen for diabetes mellitus likely will be given. Wider use of screening would likely significantly increase the numbers of commercial drivers known to have diabetes mellitus.

Terminology

The terms used to describe the different diabetic states are somewhat confusing, particularly since the older terms persist in common use and the conference reports mostly use the older terms [11,15]. Therefore, a brief review of the terms is presented. Type 1 and type 2 diabetes mellitus are the terms that will be used primarily in this chapter because they communicate the physiology of the patients [1]. Patients with type 1 diabetes mellitus are always insulin deficient and are also prone to ketoacidosis. For such individuals, insulin administration is a necessity for sustenance of life; they are truly insulin dependent. Patients with

Table 8-3.   Criteria for the diagnosis of diabetes mellitus

Diabetes mellitus	Impaired fasting glucose/glucose intolerance
1. Fasting plasma glucose > 126 mg/dL	1. Fasting plasma glucose 111–125 mg/dL
2. Two-hour oral glucose tolerance test Plasma glucose > 200 mg/dL	2. Two-hour oral glucose tolerance test Plasma glucose 140–199 mg/dL
3. Symptoms of diabetes and random plasma glucose > 200 mg/dL	

Source: American Diabetes Association, 1999.

Table 8-4. Screening criteria for diabetes mellitus

1. Age > 45 years. Screen every 3 years.

2. More frequent screening or beginning at younger ages if:
   Obese (body mass index > 27 kg/m²)
   First-degree relative affected
   High-risk ethnicity (African, Hispanic, Asian, Pacific Islander, or Native American)
   Greater than 9-lb birth weight or history of gestation diabetes
   Hypertension (>140/90 mm Hg)
   High-density lipoprotein cholesterol < 35 mg/dL or triglycerides > 250 mg/dL
   Intermediate glucose values on prior testing

Source: Adapted from American Diabetes Association, 1999.

type 2 diabetes mellitus have adequate to high levels of endogenous circulating insulin but do not use it properly. They may or may not need to administer exogenous insulin to attain improved glycemic control. Insulin-using type 2 diabetics are widely but somewhat misleadingly labeled as insulin dependent.

Insulin-dependent diabetes mellitus is the term that continues to be used in practice to describe anyone using insulin, whether type 1 or type 2. Non–insulin-dependent diabetes mellitus is the term used to describe a type 2 diabetic, but only if he or she is not being treated with insulin. The other term used in the Department of Transportation (DOT) conference reports, and thus necessarily used in this chapter, is insulin-taking diabetes mellitus (ITDM)—a term technically denoting anyone using insulin, whether type 1 or type 2, but presumably primarily dealing with type 2 insulin-using diabetics.

Screening and Diabetic Management

Commercial driver medical examinations involve two main screening elements for diabetes mellitus: one historical question ("diabetes or elevated blood sugar") and a urinalysis (glucosuria). However, many individuals who unknowingly have diabetes mellitus may go undetected by urinalysis performed for the commercial driver medical examination owing to variable thresholds for glucosuria.

The FMCSA regulations require that a diabetic driver must have the disease under "good control" and prohibit the use of insulin for interstate truck driving. There is neither a definition of good control for these purposes nor regulatory guidance of same. However, in some states, such drivers could be considered qualified to drive school buses or intrastate trucks, and the physician may still have to deal with this issue in a local jurisdiction. If a person has type 2 diabetes mellitus and the disease is controlled with diet and/or oral hypoglycemic agents, then the diabetes is not a disqualifying condition. Aspects to consider in making a determination of fitness for duty include the number and frequency of hypoglycemic reactions, the severity of the reactions, the driver's knowledge of diabetes mellitus (particularly regarding hypoglycemic risk factors and management of symptoms), and complications of the disorder. For example, for a person who has frequent hypoglycemic reactions without adequate warning of those reactions, the risk is likely too great to be allowed to drive. Thus, the physician may still judge the diabetic on oral agents as unfit to drive.

The management of diabetes mellitus is continuing to undergo significant changes. The two basic changes are (1) the switch from traditional oral hypoglycemic agents to newer pharmaceutical agents with less hypoglycemic risk and (2) tightness of control. Long-acting sulfonylureas have been prescribed for many years. These have assisted patients in maintaining compliance with medication regimens because of the infrequent dosing intervals; however, they also may result in more frequent and prolonged hypoglycemic episodes. This presents a risk for a driver who is on an unusually long haul and cannot eat at the prescribed time, as might be precipitated by unanticipated traffic or adverse weather. Other medications have been introduced in the United States (Table 8-5) and include metformin which decreases production of glucose and increases uptake. Diabetic drivers who are required to do substantial manual unloading of trucks may not be good candidates for metformin use, however, because the medication infrequently causes potentially fatal lactic acidosis, and this risk is believed to be increased in the face of vigorous activity or renal insufficiency. α-Glucosidase inhibitors have been introduced recently, and they delay absorption of glucose from the gastrointestinal tract via enzymatic blockade. Use of the α-glucosidase inhibitors as monotherapy is believed to have little risk for precipitating hypoglycemia. The thiazolidinediones assist in the management of diabetes mellitus by reducing a person's resistance to insulin. Repaglinide is thought to have less potential for precipitating hypoglycemia than the sulfonylureas. While the risk for hypoglycemia from the nonsulfonylureas is believed to range from none to low, these medications are being used in various combination therapies, and the risk for hypoglycemia in such circumstances is thought to be mildly elevated.

Table 8-5. Oral medications for type 2 diabetes mellitus*

Sulfonylureas	Alpha-glucosidase inhibitor
First generation	Acarbose (Precose)
Acetohexamide (Dymelor)	Miglitol (Glyset)
Chlorpropamide (Diabinese)	
Tolazamide (Tolinase)	**Thiazolidinediones**
Tolbutamide (Orinase)	Troglitazone (Rezulin)
Second generation	Rosiglitazone (Avandia)
Glimepiride (Amaryl)	Pioglitazone (Actos)
Glipizide (Glucotrol)	**Meglitinides**
Glyburide (DiaBeta, Micronase,	
Glynase)	Nateglinide (starlix)
Biguanide	Repaglinide (Prandin)
Metformin (Glucophage)	
Metformin/Glyburide	

*Adapted from *The Medical Letter* 2001;43(1101):29.

It is important that the examiner assess the medication regimen of the diabetic driver. The more intensive ("tight") the control with medications, the higher the likelihood for hypoglycemia.

It was believed previously that intensive control of glucose levels did not result in improved clinical outcomes. However, there now is evidence from several controlled clinical trials that intensive control does result in fewer problems with diabetic peripheral neuropathy (60 percent reduction), diabetic proliferative retinopathy (75 percent reduction at 6.5 years), diabetic nephropathy (60 percent reduction), as well as nerve conduction velocity [13,14]. Unfortunately, the major drawback of intensive control has been an increased risk for hypoglycemic reactions (threefold increased risk of severe hypoglycemic reactions). The evidence shows that individuals with intensive control are involved in more motor vehicle accidents, including deaths. While these studies were of people utilizing insulin, it would seem likely that similar results, though less stark, would apply to people on oral hypoglycemic agents attempting intensive control of glucose levels and glycohemoglobin levels.

The conflict for a commercial driver between minimizing the risk for end-organ dysfunctions via intensive control versus the risk for hypoglycemic complications continues to grow, though the increasing use of newer oral agents helps to mitigate this for those drivers who can attain control with those medications.

Assessing the Diabetic Driver

Hypoglycemic symptoms should be ascertained during the commercial driver examination process. Severe hypoglycemic events include those during which there are (1) seizures, (2) loss of consciousness, (3) hospitalizations, or (4) when the patient needs the help of another to recover (e.g., if someone else is required to retrieve a glucose source and place it in the patient's mouth).

The tightness of control also should be ascertained. This can be done by asking questions about medication regimens, goals for treatment, and hypoglycemic symptoms. Ideally, this also should be combined with recall of glycohemoglobin measurement (or records). The current target for all patients is glycohemoglobin levels less than 7 percent (still there is an elevated risk for retinopathy in those with glycohemoglobin levels of 6–7 percent) [1]. Ideally, most diabetics should know their glycohemoglobin measurement because it is a critical variable in assessing control. Yet, once they cannot address such a question, they are more likely to know the answer in the future if asked at serial examinations. These pieces of information assist the examiner in independently inferring the intensiveness of control and management of the condition. Knowledge of these issues also assists in gauging future risk for adverse events that are known to have dose-response relationships between glycemic levels and development of adverse conditions (e.g., myocardial infarction, neuropathy, retinopathy, and nephropathy).

It is recommended by the conference report on diabetic disorders and commercial drivers that the diabetic driver be evaluated by his or her personal physician at least every 6 months, although complete recertification at that time is not believed to be required [15]. Ophthalmologic examination, or at least a careful eye examination by the primary physician, also should be performed. Neurologic status should be assessed with the goal of ascertaining the presence or absence of a significant neuropathy. An electrocardiogram (ECG) is recommended at least every 2 years.

The following is a summary of the recommendations for the physical examination in a type 2 diabetic driver:

1. A focused history asking these questions:
   a. Is a hypoglycemic agent being used? Is insulin being used?
   b. Are there hypoglycemic symptoms?
   c. Does the driver have a basic knowledge of diabetes, including the effects of missed meals, particularly while taking oral hypoglycemic agents?

    d. Does the driver carry a readily accessible glucose source in the vehicle?

    e. Is the glycemic control good or at least acceptable?

    f. Does the patient self-monitor glucose levels as recommended by the conference report?

2. Physical examination that includes
    a. Neurologic assessment searching for end-organ dysfunction
    b. Retinal examination, especially if eye care is suboptimal. A careful eye examination by the primary care physician was recommended by the conference report.

3. ECG every 2 years.

4. Evaluations by the primary care physician every 6 months.

Type 2 diabetics on insulin are handled differently and are not currently considered able to drive in interstate commerce in the United States. The exceptions are those who applied for and were accepted into the diabetic waiver program (see the "Diabetes Mellitus Waivers" section). An infrequent clinical problem that occurs is the patient who is taken off insulin just prior to the examination and then placed back on the insulin after the examination and is allowed to drive. It is recommended that such individuals be considered unfit to drive interstate commercial vehicles due to lack of good control of the diabetes.

Complications of hyperglycemia include fatigue and somnolence. An individual who is poorly controlled with an oral hypoglycemic agent at the time of evaluation for commercial driver recertification also should be considered unfit for duty. He or she should be told to see his or her personal physician to get the diabetes under better control, and the certification should be withheld pending better control.

Several factors are likely to increase the risk of hypoglycemia (Table 8-6). A number of these factors apply specifically to diabetic drivers of commercial vehicles, particularly age, erratic oral intake, variability in medication schedules, and irregular sleep schedules. There also are a number of medications that place the diabetic driver at greater risk for hypoglycemic events. It is recommended that these factors and agents be evaluated carefully in a diabetic truck driver undergoing a recertification examination.

An additional complication of diabetes mellitus is retinopathy. Estimates are that 10 to 20 percent of blindness in adults is due to diabetes mellitus and that the risk estimates are 50- to 80-fold [16]. The prevalence of retinopathy is 0 percent at baseline for type 1 diabetics but approximately 18 percent for type 2 diabetics. By 15 years,

Table 8-6.   Hypoglycemia risk factors

General	Medications
Age	Long-acting oral hypoglycemic agents
Renal disease	Aspirin
Hepatic disease	Sulfa medications
Congestive heart failure	Phenylbutazone
Alcohol	Dicumarol
Irregular exercise	Chloramphenicol
Irregular meals	Beta-blockers
	Irregular medication regimens

approximately 50 percent of both groups have retinopathy [17]. Screening and laser treatment are estimated to significantly reduce the risk of blindness, including at baseline, for those with type 2 diabetes mellitus [17–20]. These data suggest additional lines of inquiry during the certification process.

Diabetes Mellitus Waivers

The U.S. FHWA experimented with a waiver program for insulin-using commercial drivers [21–24]. No new drivers are being admitted into this program, and fewer than 100 such drivers remain in the program. The driver who needs insulin is disqualified from interstate commercial vehicle operations at the current time. However, the program is being evaluated, and either waivers or exemptions may be reinstated in the future if these drivers are found to be safe. The FHWA convened a panel of experts in the late 1980s and obtained an opinion that people who take insulin can and do drive safely as long as some fairly stringent requirements are met [11]. As a result, the FHWA began to enroll people in this waiver program and another waiver program for vision. Approximately 139 diabetics were initially certified before a court injunction that stopped further enrollments was obtained at the request of a trade group [21]. It was argued that the program was not proven to be safe and that studies had shown diabetics to have an elevated risk for accidents. Those people who obtained the waivers were allowed to continue, but new enrollments were stopped [21]. Information on the accident rates of the drivers operating with diabetic waivers to date has not shown an elevated risk in this select group. A recent publication from the FHWA indicated that the accident rate in the waiver group was 2.31 per million vehicle miles traveled ($n = 13$) compared with the national rate of 2.61 ($n = 444,000$). The property damage rate was lower in the waiver group (1.78 versus 2.05), the injury rate was the same for both (0.53), and the fatality rate was lower (0.00 versus 0.03). Problems with these data are that they involve small numbers, the program was nonrandom/uncontrolled, the drivers with waivers were required to have had a good driving record for the prior 3 years, and the comparison population was not truly comparable. This last problem is probably an underrecognized problem with these data. The comparison population included people who likely have disqualifying or poorly controlled conditions but who have been given licenses by those who do not know the regulations. For a valid comparison to assess the hazards of insulin use in truck drivers, it would seem that the comparison population also should have been under similar scrutiny.

The requirements for inclusion in the diabetes waiver program included

1. Five years' experience as a truck driver

2. A clean driving record

3. No history of having complications or diabetic ketoacidosis

4. Regular follow-up

5. A careful commercial driver history and physical examination

6. An endocrinology evaluation within 2 months of the commercial driver exam (The evaluation was to review that the patient had passed a diabetic education program and reviewed use of a glucose log and to document that the patient was free of complications, free of diabetic reactions, and willing to manage the diabetes.)

7. Ophthalmologic, neurologic, and cardiovascular examinations

This information is reviewed in detail for reasons that both the concepts of how to handle diabetics may be more widely applicable and the probability that exemptions will be given in the future with similar requirements is considered fairly likely.

The requirements for a driver granted a diabetes waiver included the following:

1. The driver was required to carry a readily absorbable source of glucose.

2. The driver was required to carry a glucose meter that contains a memory function. This was required, in part, so that if there was an accident, a prompt glucose measurement could be retrieved.

3. The driver was required to maintain logs.

4. Finger-stick glucose measurements were required 1 hour before and every 4 hours while driving.

5. Even minor infractions have to be reported, not just those as routinely required by the DOT.

6. The DOT card had to state "Medically qualified by operation of 49 CFR 391.64."

7. Logs had to be submitted on request, including those of the glucose measurements.

Assumptions made by the panels of experts for the DOT conference reports seemed reasonable at the time but no longer seem so secure. Yet these assumptions have been the basis for action at the Federal level. They include the following (information in parentheses indicates currently contrasting issues):

1. The number of people in the United States with diabetes mellitus has been assumed to be relatively stable. (However, since the prevalence of obesity is rising, job tasks are becoming more sedentary, and screening for diabetes mellitus is now recommended, this assumption is invalid.)

2. The percentage of people taking insulin will be stable. (This is also not a reliable assumption. In an attempt to have more people on intensive regimens, there may be more people who begin to use insulin. Alternatively, with more oral medications, it is possible that some diabetics who are not on large doses of insulin may be able to switch to oral regimens. Last, if any of the weight loss medications were ever successful on a sustained basis, the number of people on insulin would likely decrease rather than rise.)

3. The number of severe reactions per year will be stable. (As noted earlier, the number of severe reactions is likely quite unstable now, particularly with the advent and wider adoption of intensive regimens.)

Thus, diabetes is an ever-challenging management problem, particularly in the setting of commercial driving. While there are very few drivers currently operating in interstate commerce with insulin/diabetic waivers, it is quite possible that exemptions for select drivers will be implemented in the future. This will add to the challenges of performing commercial driver medical examinations.

Diabetes, Hypoglycemia, and Accident Risk

Studies of the accident risk from diabetes mellitus present somewhat conflicting results and are also very difficult to evaluate due to heterogeneity of the data. There is usually a lack of stratification of drivers in analytical studies into treatment categories by diet, traditional oral agents, newer oral agents (lower risk for hypoglycemia), insulin, and combinations of treatment that would be particularly meaningful in the commercial medical examination process. Further useful distinctions of intensive versus usual control are also nearly always absent.

Insulin-using type 2 diabetic truck drivers enrolled in a program with very stringent criteria were found not to have an elevated accident rate compared with the entire population of commercial vehicle drivers [12]. A study of those same data by the Federal Motor Carrier Safety Administration concluded that insulin users did not have an elevated risk [21]. Those results were similar to a study of Quebec diabetic truck driver crash risks [25].

Yet a study of German truck drivers found elevated odds ratios (ORs) for symptomatic hypoglycemia attributed to insulin use compared with those treated with oral agents, whether treated with conventional insulin (OR = 1.8), intensive insulin (OR = 3.7), or insulin pumps (OR = 4.6) [26]. Additionally, a randomized controlled experimental study found evidence for impairments at mild degrees of hypoglycemia, 59.4–72 mg/dL (3.3 to 4.0 mmol/L), and most of the drivers did not take corrective action while performing driving simulations [27], while another study found decrements in performance at 64.8 mg/dL (3.6 mmol/L) [28].

A 5-year population-based study in the State of Utah found that the risk for all motor vehicle drivers with diabetes was elevated whether on restrictions (relative risk [RR] = 1.38, 95% CI = 0.75–2.54) or not restricted (RR = 1.30, 95% CI = 1.23–1.38). At-fault motor vehicle crash risks were similarly nonsignificant but elevated for those on restrictions (RR = 1.77, 95% CI = 0.87–3.61) but statistically significant for those not restricted (RR = 1.48, 95% CI = 1.36–1.58) [29]. Most, but not all, studies have found similar results [30–36]. Last, when those with diabetes mellitus also have other disorders (e.g., cardiovascular disease), there seem to be generally more consistent studies and higher estimates of risk [29,30]. One of the challenges in this area is the determination of safety based upon objective criteria, as most of the criteria for granting of licensure are at least somewhat subjective and thus able to be influenced by the prospective driver.

In summary, there are significant conflicts among a person's right to drive, a person's right to earn a living, society's acceptance of a reasonable level of risk to other drivers, an acceptable level of risk to children in a school bus, a person's health status, the needs of families, an acceptable level of risk for employers, and medical judgment. There continues to be a chasm of silence to the answer to this conundrum.

Thyroid Disorders

Thyroid disorders are common endocrine system abnormalities with a prevalence estimated at 1 to 4 percent of adults [37]. Increasing age and female gender are two prominent risk factors. The annual incidence of hypothyroid states is slightly higher than that for hyperthyroid states. Data on motor vehicle crash risks are absent. Generally, these problems are believed to be unlikely to interfere with an individual's ability to drive because they usually present in a mild state. However, there are some exceptions.

An individual with significant symptoms of thyrotoxicosis or "thyroid storm" would best be temporarily deferred from recertification. In addition, a driver with profound hypothyroidism should not be recertified until the disease manifestations are brought under reasonable control, often after a month or more. However, most patients with hypothyroidism develop the symptoms slowly and notice weight gain; recertification of such patients probably should not be withheld. If there is any concern about the patient's willingness or ability to maintain the prescribed medical regimen, a short recertification, for a few weeks to 3 months, can be given. On achieving a stable medical regimen, the driver can be returned to a standard 2-year recertification interval.

In Australia, there are no specific recommendations. "Endocrine disorders with symptoms which could affect the ability to drive a vehicle safely should be individually assessed" [emphasis added] [10].

In Canada, the Canadian Medical Association recommends that those with "hyperthyroidism complicated by cardiac or neurologic symptoms should not drive any type of motor vehicle until the condition has been controlled [9]." Those with symptomatic hypothyroidism also are believed not to be candidates to drive until the condition is controlled successfully. Parathyroid disorders also are addressed, and it is recommended that "patients who have parathyroid conditions with increased muscle weakness or muscular excitability should not be allowed to drive." There are no detailed guidelines for thyroid disorders. Thus, these situations are left to the examiner's judgment. It may be best for the examiner to ask himself or herself a question such as, "Is this person able to drive safely?" or "Would I like to have this person on the road next to me?" Because most people are reasonable, asking the driver such questions may prompt quick understanding and agreement that he or she should defer driving until better able to do so safely.

Hypothalamic-Pituitary-Adrenocortical Axis Disorders

These endocrine disorders parallel those of the thyroid in that they generally do not prevent re-certification. Often, these disorders are slow in onset. If symptoms are severe, however, such as severe Addison's disease, then FHWA re-certification should be withheld until the disorder is brought under better control. In contrast, the Canadian Medical Examination seems to recommend that patients with diabetes insipidus, Addison's disease, acromegaly (with complicating factors) or untreated Cushing's syndrome not be allowed to drive commercial vehicles [9]. Similar to thyroid disorders, there is no specific guidance in Australia [10].

References

1. American Diabetes Association. Report of the expert committee on the diagnosis and classification of diabetes mellitus. *Diabetes Care* 2000;23(Suppl. 1):S4–S19.
2. Harris MI, Flegal KM, Cowie CC, et al. Prevalence of diabetes, impaired fasting glucose, and impaired glucose tolerance in U.S. adults. *Diabetes Care* 1998;21:518–524.
3. American Diabetes Association. National Diabetes Fact Sheet, 2000. *http://www.diabetes.org/main/info/facts/facts_natl.jsp*. Accessed Dec. 18, 2002.

4. Harris MI. Prevalence of non–insulin-dependent diabetes and impaired glucose tolerance. In: National Diabetes Data Group, ed. *Diabetes in America: Diabetes Data Compiled 1984.* Washington: U.S. Department of Health and Human Services, 1985:VI1–VI31.

5. DiaMond Project Group on Social Issues. Global regulations on diabetics treated with insulin and their operation of commercial motor vehicles. *BMJ* 1993;307(6898):250–253.

6. Qualification of drivers; exemption applications; diabetes. *Fed Reg* 2001;66(July 31):39548–39553.

7. Gill G, Durston J, Johnston R, MacLeod K, Watkins P. Insulin-treated diabetes and driving in the UK. *Diabet Med* 2002;19:435–439.

8. Driver and Vehicle Licensing Agency. At-a-Glance Guide to the Current Medical Standards of Fitness to Drive. Swansea, England: Drivers Medical Unit, DVLA. *http://www.dvla.gov.uk/at_a_glance/content.htm.* Accessed Dec. 9, 2002.

9. Canadian Medical Association. Physicians' Guide to Driver Examination. Ottawa, Canada. *http://www.cma.ca/cma/common/displayPage.do?pageld=/staticContent/HTML/publications/catalog/driversguide/index.htm.* Accessed Dec. 9, 2002.

10. Australasian Faculty of Occupational Medicine. Medical Examinations of Commercial Vehicle Drivers. Prepared for the National Road Transport Commission and the Federal Office of Road Safety, Sydney, Australia, 1997. *http://www.nrtc.gov.au/publications/assessment.pdf.* Accessed Dec. 9, 2002.

11. U.S. Department of Transportation, Federal Highway Administration. *Insulin-Using Commercial Motor Vehicle Drivers.* Publication No. FHWA-MC-92-012. Washington: U.S. DOT, Federal Highway Administration, Office of Motor Carriers, 1992.

12. U.S. Preventive Services Task Force. Screening for diabetes mellitus. In: *Guide to Clinical Preventive Services,* 2nd ed. Baltimore: Williams & Wilkins, 1996.

13. The Diabetes Control and Complications Trial Research Group. The effect of intensive treatment of diabetes on the development and progression of long-term complications in insulin-dependent diabetes mellitus. *N Engl J Med* 1993;329:977–986.

14. Reichard P, Nilsson B-Y, Rosenqvist U. The effect of long-term intensified insulin treatment on the development of microvascular complications of diabetes mellitus. *N Engl J Med* 1993;329:304–309.

15. U.S. Department of Transportation, Federal Highway Administration. *Conference on Diabetic Disorders and Commercial Drivers.* Publication No. FHWA-MC-88-041. Washington: U.S. DOT, Federal Highway Administration, Office of Motor Carriers, 1988.

16. Sjolie AK, Green A. Blindness in insulin treated diabetic patients with age at onset < 30 years. *J Chronic Dis* 1987;40:215–220.

17. Kristinsson JK, Hauksdottir H, Stefánsson E, Jonasson F, Gislason I. Active prevention in diabetic eye disease. *Acta Ophthalmol Scand* 1997;75:249–254.

18. Early Treatment Diabetic Retinopathy Research Study Group. Photocoagulation for diabetic macular edema: ETDRS report number 1. *Arch Ophthalmol* 1985;103:1796–1806.

19. Klein R, Klein BE, Moss SE, Davis MD, DeMets DL. The Wisconsin Epidemiological Study of Diabetic Retinopathy, IX: Four-year incidence and progression of diabetic retinopathy when age at diagnosis is less than 30 years. *Arch Ophthalmol* 1989;107:237–243.

20. Klein R, Klein BE, Moss SE, Davis MD, DeMets DL. The Wisconsin Epidemiological Study of Diabetic Retinopathy, X: Four-year incidence and progression of diabetic retinopathy when age at diagnosis is 30 years or more. *Arch Ophthalmol* 1989;107:244–249.

21. U.S. Department of Transportation, Federal Motor Carrier Safety Administration. An analysis of the risks associated with the operation of commercial motor vehicles by drivers with insulin-treated diabetes mellitus concluded that they were not at elevated risk. FMCSA-PPD-02-001. Washington: U.S. DOT, Federal Motor Carrier Safety Administration, 2001.

22. Qualifications of drivers: Vision and diabetes—limited exemptions. *Fed Reg* 1996;61(March 26):13338–13347.

23. Qualifications of drivers: Vision and diabetes—proposed rule. *Fed Reg* 1996;61(Jan. 8):606–611.

24. Qualification of drivers: Waivers—diabetes. *Fed Reg* 1993;58(July 29):40690–40697.

25. Laberge-Nadeau C, Desjardins D, Dionne G, et al. Impact of diabetes on crash risks of truck-permit holders and commercial drivers. *Diabetes Care* 2000;23:612–617.

26. Harsch IA, Stocker S, Radespiel-Troger M, et al. Traffic hypoglycaemias and accidents in patients with diabetes mellitus treated with different antidiabetic regimens. *J Intern Med* 2002;252:352–360.

27. Cox DJ, Gonder-Frederick LA, Kovatchev BP, Julian DM, Clark WL. Progressive hypoglycemia's impact on driving simulation performance. *Diabetes Care* 2000;23:163–170.

28. Cox D, Clarke W, Gonder-Frederick L, Kovatchev B. Driving mishaps and hypoglycemia: Risk and prevention. *Int J Clin Pract* 2001;123(suppl.):38–42.

29. Diller E, Cook L, Leonard D, Reading J, Dean JM, Vernon D. Evaluating drivers licensed with medical conditions in Utah, 1992–1996. NHTSA Technical Report DOT HS 809 023. Washington: National Highway Traffic Safety Administration, June 1999.

30. Koepsell TD, Wolf ME, McCloskey L, et al. Medical conditions and motor vehicle collision injuries in older adults. *J Am Geriatr Soc* 1994;42(7):695–700.

31. Gerard D. The effect of intensive treatment of diabetes mellitus [letter]. *N Engl J Med* 1994;330:642.

32. Hansotia P. Seizure disorders, diabetes mellitus and cerebrovascular disease: Considerations for older drivers. *Clin Geriatr Med* 1993;9(2):323–339.

33. Hansotia P, Broste S. The effects of epilepsy and diabetes mellitus on the risk of automobile accidents. *N Engl J Med* 1991;324:22–26.

34. Marottoli RA, Cooney LM Jr, Wagner DR, et al. Predictors of automobile crashes and moving violations among elderly drivers. *Ann Intern Med* 1994;121(11):842–846.

35. Waller JA. Chronic medical conditions and traffic safety. *N Engl J Med* 1965;273(26):1413–1420.

36. Ysander L. The safety of drivers with chronic disease. *Br J Ind Med* 1966;23:28–36.

37. Office of Motor Carrier Research and Standards. *Qualification of Drivers—Vision and Diabetes.* Tech Brief, Publication No. FHWA-MCRT-99-017. Washington: U.S. Department of Transportation, Federal Highway Administration, September 1999.

9

Psychiatric Disorders

Kurt T. Hegmann, MD, MPH

The lack of quality data on accident risks combined with nonspecific advisory criteria make the assessment of drivers with psychiatric disorders regarding fitness to drive commercial vehicles a challenging problem for the examining doctor [1].

The risks of motor vehicle crashes among those with psychiatric disorders are not well defined. Data on commercial drivers are absent.

Some data from the general driving population are available. It has been shown that a history of mental illness conferred about a twofold increased risk of accidents (15.3 versus 7.2 accidents per 1 million miles) [2]. Comparable results were found in a 5-year population-based study that demonstrated elevated risks for motor vehicle crashes among those with psychiatric or emotional conditions whether on restrictions (relative risk [RR] = 1.87, 95% confidence interval [CI] = 1.11–3.17) or unrestricted (RR = 1.57, 95% CI = 1.46–1.67) [3]. Those drivers were at still higher risk for at-fault motor vehicle crashes whether on restrictions (RR = 2.98, 95% CI = 1.64–5.07) or unrestricted (RR = 1.85, 95% CI = 1.69–2.01). Also, from that same study, those with learning, memory, or communication problems were at about twice the risk for motor vehicle crashes and more than threefold the risk for at-fault crashes.

Far more data are available regarding the risks of psychoactive medication use and the general driving population's motor vehicle crash rates than those for disease states. Most of those data concern increased risks associated with use of benzodiazepines, barbiturates, opioids, and antidepressants [4–12].

Psychiatric Disorders and the CDME Certification Process

Requirements

There are no specific, mandatory psychiatric criteria. However, there are many disorders, conditions, and medication uses that are recommended for disqualification by the conference report [13].

Recommendations

The procedure proposed by the U.S. Department of Transportation (DOT) conference report on psychiatric disorders [13] for handling psychiatric problems was similar to that recommended by the conference report on neurologic disorders (Table 9-1). The procedure would likely work with virtually any medical problem and organ system.

Although the mechanism proposed in the conference report has not been implemented, it provides a valuable framework for handling psychiatric problems; however, one caveat should be kept in mind: The conference report "strongly" recommended a neurologic, psychiatric, or neuropsychological evaluation for any central nervous system (CNS) problem or medical condition that has the potential to cause CNS damage or in anyone with a family history of a degenerative neurologic disorder. As written, this is an impractical recommendation owing to the number of referrals required and the poor likelihood ratio for that approach. It is probably more appropriate to refer individuals with

---

Table 9-1. Commercial driver medical examination guidelines for psychiatric disorders*

1. Commercial driver medical examination reveals a problem.

2. Referral to a psychiatrist, neurologist, or neuropsychologist to confirm *DSM-IV* diagnosis; some are disqualified at this step.

3. Neuropsychological or other psychometric testing may be performed; some are disqualified at this step.

4. A road test may be done to confirm the ability to drive.

---

*Adapted from the Conference on Psychiatric Disorders and Commercial Drivers [13].

mildly active psychiatric problems for consideration of their ability to drive. If there is a substantially active problem, then a referral is probably unnecessary because the person is not likely to be qualified to drive. Referral to an appropriate individual to confirm the American Psychiatric Association's *Diagnostic and Statistical Manual, 4th Edition (DSM-IV)* diagnosis and a joint determination of whether to disqualify the individual is likely needed in uncertain circumstances. Neuropsychological evaluation and tests may be ordered as well, depending on the situation. The conference report notes that no data or little data exist for many disorders, and thus the report is a summation of "educated guesses" and recommendations from a panel of experts.

Great Britain handles psychiatric problems in a somewhat similar manner. Drivers with relapsing, recurrent, or progressive psychiatric disorders are required to be reported and investigated [14].

Psychotropic Medications

Many psychiatric patients take multiple medications simultaneously ("polypharmacy"). This may present additional problems in evaluations, but it may also simplify other cases as signifying higher risk and likelihood of disqualification. An observational but uncontrolled study failed to confirm the impression that individuals taking selective serotonin reuptake inhibitors (SSRIs) are more likely to perform better on tests such as reaction times; instead, only 11.4 percent were believed to have passed all tests administered, and there were no differences between SSRIs, monoamine oxidase inhibitors (MAOIs), and tricyclic antidepressants [15]. Although definitive disqualification of such complex prospective drivers is not delineated in the conference report, these data and other information suggest that those requiring multiple medications to control psychiatric problems deserve at least an additional opinion, if not outright disqualification, as an inference on severity of the problems.

Benzodiazepines have been associated with an elevated risk for motor vehicle accidents in a number of studies. Of further concern is one study by Barbone and colleagues [4] that also showed a similarly increased risk for short-acting medications. The risk for minor tranquilizer use has been estimated to be as high as 4.9, although most studies have found much smaller estimates of elevated risk.

One other group of medications to be mentioned is the antihistamines, since these are occasionally prescribed as anxiolytics. They have long been thought to be sedating and thus place a driver at increased risk of motor vehicle accidents. Some reports have drawn this association [7–10]. Newer, selective antihistamines for allergies are thought to be less sedating, yet there also is a study by O'Hanlon and Ramaekers [9] that shows some sedating effects of the newer antihistamine agents on measures of driver performance.

The Australasian Faculty of Occupational Medicine statement regarding psychoactive medications states, "More than for perhaps any other category of medical condition, careful individual assessments need to be made of commercial vehicle drivers using psychoactive drugs" [1]. An individualized approach was recommended for most psychiatric conditions.

The Canadian Medical Association (CMA) has written that "Physicians who prescribe drugs known to have an effect on sensory, mental or physical functions have a clear responsibility to warn their patients that these drugs may affect their ability to drive safely" [16].

The conference report recommends that use of a number of medications should result in disqualification (Table 9-2). When dealing with an examinee who uses one or more of these medications, the commercial driver medical examiner likely will need to send the driver to a psychiatrist to determine whether he or she can drive safely, since most commercial driver medical examiners are unlikely to routinely prescribe these medications for psychiatric conditions and, as such, are unlikely to be familiar with their effects. The conference report recommends that use of benzodiazepines for anxiolytic purposes, use of tricyclic antidepressants, and use of barbiturates should be disqualifying. The only exception noted is that an individual who is treated effectively with nonsedating anxiolytics such as buspirone may be qualified. Individuals who require hypnotics were recommended to use, under medical supervision, only short-acting drugs with half-lives of less than 5 hours for no more than 2 weeks. If a patient is stable on lithium, he or she may be qualified. Again, however, most commercial driver medical examiners are not likely to be familiar with lithium or the evaluation of bipolar disorder patients and probably would need the assistance of a psychiatrist to judge the driving abilities of most such patients. Antidepressants are believed to be largely disqualifying medications, although it is recognized that some medications are not as sedating or impairing and that an individual taking such a medication may be qualified. The conference report recommended that there be a minimum of 3 months after electroconvulsive therapy prior to DOT certification. However, this also likely requires the judgment of a psychiatrist and an assessment of stability, including an assessment of any potential impairment from medications prescribed. Antipsychotic

Table 9-2. Psychiatric medications and conditions*

Disqualifying	May be qualified†
Benzodiazepines	Buspirone
Hypnotics	Short-acting hypnotics and < 2 weeks' use
Barbiturates	
Tricyclic antidepressants	Amitriptyline, 25 mg every night
	Fluoxetine
	Bupropion
Antipsychotics	Stable on lithium
	>3 months after electroconvulsive therapy
	Valproic acid
	Carbamazepine
Psychosis	Psychosis but symptom free > 1 year
	Anorexia nervosa
	Bulimia
	Personality disorders

*Adapted from the *Conference on Psychiatric Disorders and Commercial Drivers* [13].
†Psychiatric evaluation prior to clearance is recommended.

medications are thought to be disqualifying. Stimulants of the CNS also are believed to be disqualifying, with the possible exception of stimulants used in certain controlled situations such as narcolepsy. However, this conflicts with the conference report on neurologic disorders (see Chapter 7).

One psychoactive drug that is not well assessed with the current examination form is tobacco. Despite significant impacts on health possibly surpassed only by obesity, this is not assessed in the commercial driver certification process unless the examiner either makes specific inquiries with each driver or the clinic revises the examination form to include such question(s).

Australian criteria disqualify patients taking chronic psychoactive medications that "impair driving performance on a long-term basis" [1]. Exceptions are that there is a supportive psychiatric opinion, or the psychotic condition is "so well controlled as to reduce the risk of an exacerbation to that of any member of the general population."

Anxiety Disorders

Aside from the condition itself, there is also a concern about driver impairment from the medications used to treat anxiety disorders. As noted previously, an elevated risk of motor vehicle accidents is reported with benzodiazepine use. A list of the medications used to treat anxiety (Table 9-2) as represented in the conference report is updated in Table 9-3 [17]. Buspirone is believed to have the least sedating potential [11].

Table 9-3. Medications for anxiety and depression*

Antidepressant medications

Tricyclics
  Amitriptyline
  Desipramine
  Imipramine
  Nortriptyline
  Protripyline-Deprex
  Trimipramine

Selective serotonin reuptake
    inhibitors
  Citalopram
  Fluoxetine
  Paroxetine
  Escitalopram
  Sertraline

Monoamine oxidase inhibitors
  Phenelzine
  Tranylcypromine

Other
  Bupropion
  Mirtazapine
  Nefazodone
  Trazodone
  Amoxapine
  Venlafaxine
  Hydroxyzine
  Thioridazine

Antianxiety medications

Benzodiazepines
  Alprazolam
  Clonazepam
  Diazepam
  Lorazepam
  Chlordiazepoxide
  Doxepin
  Oxazepam
  Clorazepate

Other
  Buspirone

---

*Adapted from *Med Lett Drugs Ther* 2002;44(1140):83 [17].

Generalized anxiety disorder is believed to be potentially impairing, particularly if severe, untreated, or associated with depression, drug use, or other anxiety disorders. Psychiatric referral is recommended by the conference report, and consideration of a driving test with an occupational therapist also is recommended. Some individuals with post-traumatic stress disorder (PTSD) are believed to have a greater potential for motor vehicle accidents. With this disorder, there may be a loss of regard for personal safety, whether or not the PTSD occurred secondary to a motor vehicle accident. Psychiatric referral and consideration of a driving test were recommended. Agoraphobia warrants the same treatment. Social phobia is believed not to warrant further evaluation.

Attention Deficit Hyperactivity Disorder

The attention deficit hyperactivity disorder (ADHD) is garnering increasing attention as a problem in the adult population. Part of the reason for this interest is that individuals diagnosed as having ADHD 10 to 20 years ago are now entering the workforce. Quite a few studies that have followed these individuals over time have found an elevated risk for traffic offenses, licensure suspensions, and motor vehicle crashes [18–20]. Nearly all these studies examined only ADHD patients through approximately age 25 years. Most of the elevated risk seems to be in those who were most severely affected as children. Nevertheless, how to evaluate such a prospective commercial driver is uncertain.

Since some features of this disorder are believed to carry over into adulthood, the conference report recommended that examiners evaluating individuals with this past history do the following:

1. Arrange a practical driving test conducted by an occupational therapist.

2. Make collateral contact with employers and others who have observed the examinee in tasks requiring sustained attention.

3. Evaluate the examinee's complete legal and driving records.

4. Review a detailed work history of the examinee, with particular attention to the length of service and the reason for and mode of termination for each employer.

Depression, Bipolar, and Other Mood Disorders

Depression is a common disorder with a prevalence in the general population estimated to be 3 to 5 percent [21]. Depression also has been associated with an elevated risk for motor vehicle accidents. A study by MacPherson and colleagues [7] estimated that the risk for antidepressant use increased 4.63-fold ($p < 0.001$). On the other hand, in a study by Ray and colleagues [10] that analyzed the risk of cyclic antidepressant use by dose, no elevated risk was found for those using low doses (i.e., amitriptyline at up to 25 mg/d). Beyond this, the risk was increased approximately 2.2-fold [11]. A study of moderate to severe depression evaluating psychomotor reaction function and times in a hospitalized setting found that only 11.4 percent passed all tests administered, and there were believed to be no significant differences between those using tricyclic antidepressants, MAOIs, or SSRIs [22].

A list of these medications as updated from Table 9-2 is presented in Table 9-3. Generally, the SSRIs and the MAOIs are thought to have less sedating properties than the tricyclic antidepressants. However, fatigue is a side effect reported in excess compared with placebo for several of these medications in controlled clinical trials. Increased complaints of sedation or fatigue also were seen for nefazodone, trazodone, and mirtazapine. Also of potential concern for the commercial driver medical examiner are the side effects of agitation, anxiety, and insomnia that may occur with bupropion [17], as well as similar effects with use of some of the other medications.

The conference report recommended that drivers with histories of depression, bipolar disorder, and other mood disorders be evaluated by a psychiatrist. Any actively manic, suicidal, or severely depressed individual should not be qualified. Symptoms from severe depression, mania, or a suicide attempt would need to be absent for at least 1 year prior to recertification. All drivers without active disease but with a history of these disorders were recommended to be evaluated every 2 years by a psychiatrist.

The CMA recommends that "If the physician believes that a patient's judgment or psychomotor activity has been severely affected by his or her emotional state, the patient should be advised not to drive any type of motor vehicle until sufficiently recovered. The possible side effects of any prescribed drugs should be considered when making this assessment" [16].

In Great Britain, drivers with minor anxiety or depression are believed to be capable of being certified, and no notification of the driver licensing agency is necessary [14]. However, more severe states are believed to not be certifiable until stable for 6 months. Australian guidelines are the same as those for schizophrenia noted earlier [1].

Dissociative Disorders

Individuals with multiple personality disorder are believed to need psychiatric evaluation and a driving test. However, it is difficult to envision a situation in which such a person could be considered qualified. Individuals with psychogenic fugue, psychogenic amnesia, and depersonalization need psychiatric evaluation and further investigation, particularly with respect to their driving record.

Eating Disorders

Eating disorders and personality disorders are mentioned in the conference report as being possibly disqualifying conditions depending on the situation. It was recommended that a psychiatrist evaluate all individuals with a history of these disorders. Patients with active eating disorders should be disqualified. Those with significant malnutrition or fluid/electrolyte disturbances from these disorders were recommended to be stable for 1 year prior to consideration for recertification. All individuals with a past history of these problems were believed to require evaluation every 2 years by a psychiatrist.

Factitious Disorder

Those with factitious disorder should be evaluated carefully because they may engage in behaviors that are very risky in the commercial driving business, such as injecting insulin to induce hypoglycemia, thus attaining the role of the sick. Any active factitious disorder was believed to require psychiatric evaluation, although a remote and inactive problem is believed not to require further evaluation.

Personality Disorders

Drivers with personality disorders are thought to have an elevated accident risk [1]. In Australia, such persons are to be "managed through administrative channels. Their fitness to drive—on personality criteria alone—is not considered to be a medical decision" [1].

The personality disorders considered in the DOT conference report included paranoid, schizoid, schizotypal, antisocial, borderline histrionic, narcissistic, avoidant, dependent, obsessive-compulsive, and passive-aggressive personality disorders. Individuals with histrionic, narcissistic, and dependent personality disorders were not recommended for special evaluations. Those with obsessive-compulsive and passive-aggressive disorders were thought to be somewhat intermediate, with a potential to have an increased risk for motor vehicle accidents. Those diagnosed as having obsessive-compulsive disorder should be asked questions to assess the degree of excess hostility, aggressive tendencies, vulnerability to stress, and past job dysfunction to evaluate the need for further assessment. Passive-aggressive traits deemed worthy of further investigation include recent suicidal or homicidal thoughts, hospitalization in the past 6 months, or a history of arrest for a violent offense. The general approach recommended for evaluating the other problems includes an assessment to confirm accuracy of the diagnosis, assessment of past ability to drive safely, and reliance on collateral interviews to assess the risks of allowing the individual to drive. It is noteworthy that antisocial personality disorder and alcoholism are the two psychological factors thought to most likely result in motor vehicle accidents.

Disorders of impulse control, such as intermittent explosive disorder, kleptomania, pathologic gambling, and pyromania, also were addressed. Intermittent explosive disorder is recommended to be evaluated by a psychiatrist or psychologist, with special attention being paid to hostility, violence, tolerance to stress, unsafe driving practices, school/military/employment records, and violent thought content. Other disorders of impulse control may occur in the setting of other psychological disorders or may occur in individuals with impulsive and risky behaviors that should be assessed by a psychiatrist prior to certification.

A study of "road rage" deserves mention. Although it is not a disorder, it is thought to be associated with several disorders. This study found that factors associated with road rage were male gender, history of illicit drug use, history of evaluation/treatment for emotional problems, and an inverse relationship with years of driving [23].

In Australia, those with personality disorders are generally not believed to be qualified to drive as "Such people often show disregard for social values and the law; they may have a history of aggressive, irresponsible or erratic behaviour which may be evidenced by repeated traffic violations and civil charges" [1]. In Great Britain, those with "persistent behaviour disorder" are to notify the driver license agency and generally will have the license revoked until the "person matures and psychiatric reports confirm stability. . . ." The CMA also noted that "People with personality disorders often show a wanton disregard for accepted social values and have a history of erratic, aggressive or irresponsible behaviour, which may include repeated traffic violations. Patients exhibiting these characteristics should not be allowed to drive without very careful consideration and a psychiatric assessment" [16].

Schizophrenia and Psychoses

A study of inpatients recovering from acute schizophrenic episodes and expected to be discharged within 2 weeks found that only 10.7 percent were believed to have passed a battery of psychomotor tests, whereas 32 percent were believed to have impairments requiring further evaluation of the ability to drive and 57 percent were considered severely impaired and unqualified to drive. Those treated with clozapine tended to perform better than those treated with usual neuroleptics, though the results were not always statistically significant [24].

Schizophrenia is considered to be a chronic and permanently disqualifying condition, as recommended in the DOT conference report [13]. Those with active psychoses should be prohibited from commercial vehicle operation. It was recommended that individuals be free of psychotic episodes for 1 year prior to consideration for certification. If a person had only a brief psychosis, the option for evaluating the patient 6 months after the event was noted as a possibility. The conference report also recommended reevaluation every 2 years for those whose mental illness histories have psychotic features, and such drivers were instructed to report any psychotic symptoms within 30 days. I believe that, at least initially, recertifications more frequently than every 2 years would be more appropriate and that any patient with psychotic symptoms should report symptoms on the date of occurrence.

The CMA also believes that acute psychosis is incompatible with any motor vehicle operation. Furthermore, "anyone wishing to drive passenger-carrying or commercial . . . vehicles should be free of psychotic episodes for at least 1 year and should receive a favourable assessment by a consultant. The physician should pay particular attention to any recent history of suicidal tendencies, paranoid delusions or violent and aggressive behaviour" [16].

Acute psychosis is believed to be incompatible with driving in Great Britain [14]. Those with any episode of psychosis are not believed to be able to safely drive unless there is no recurrence for at least 3 years and there is insight into the condition. Chronic schizophrenia is not believed to be incompatible with driving provided the person is stable for 3 years and has insight into his or her condition and there are no significant adverse medication effects.

Patients with acute psychosis are believed to be unqualified in Australia [1]. If a driver is no longer acutely psychotic but the examiner believes that there is a significant risk of relapse, he or she is not qualified.

Somatoform Disorders

Individuals with body dysmorphic disorder, hypochondriasis, somatization disorder, and undifferentiated somatization disorder are believed not to have difficulty driving.

Those with either conversion disorder or somatoform pain disorder are believed to have an elevated accident potential, so a psychiatric evaluation and consideration of a practical driving test with an occupational therapist are recommended.

Conclusion

In a practical light, a number of disorders discussed previously would seem unlikely to result in licensure for an applicant. Psychiatric evaluation is likely needed for prospective drivers with a number of these conditions. Regardless of the diagnosis or situation, if the commercial driver medical examiner is uncomfortable with an individual's mental aspects, a psychiatric evaluation is warranted. It is probably best to communicate with the psychiatrist prior to such a consultation. However, should the psychiatrist establish that the person can drive safely and the examiner still has lingering doubts, it is my opinion that the examiner should (1) (re)contact the psychiatrist, (2) inform him or her of the concerns, and (3) request a letter in writing from the psychiatrist stating that there is no increased risk of a motor vehicle accident with this applicant. In individuals for whom there is no such concern or in individuals with a history of a problem that has been silent for years, certification would seem to be justifiable.

References

1. Australasian Faculty of Occupational Medicine. Medical Examinations of Commercial Vehicle Drivers. Prepared for the National Road Transport Commission and the Federal Office of Road Safety. Australia, 1997. *http://www.nrtc.gov.au/publications/medd.asp?lo=public.* Accessed Dec. 9, 2002.
2. Waller JA. Chronic medical conditions and traffic safety. *N Engl J Med* 1965;273(26):1413–1420.
3. Diller E, Cook L, Leonard D, Reading J, Dean JM, Vernon D. Evaluating drivers licensed with medical conditions in Utah, 1992–1996. NHTSA Technical Report DOTHS 809 023. Washington: National Highway Traffic Safety Administration, June 1999.
4. Barbone F, McMahon AD, Davey PG, et al. Association of road-traffic accidents with benzodiazepine use. *Lancet* 1998;352:1333–1336.
5. Koepsell TD, Wolf ME, McCloskey L, et al. Medical conditions and motor vehicle collision injuries in older adults. *J Am Geriatr Soc* 1994;42(7):695–700.
6. Laux LF, Brelsford J. Age-related changes in sensory, cognitive, psychomotor and physical functioning and driving performance in drivers aged 40 to 92. Washington: AAA Foundation for Traffic Safety, 1990:1–58.
7. MacPherson RD, Perl J, Stramer GA, et al. Self-reported drug-usage and crash-incidence in breathalyzed drivers. *Accid Anal Prev* 1984;2:139–148.
8. Morris LN, Allman RM, Owsley C, et al. Vehicle crashes and positive urine drug screens among older drivers. *Clin Epidemiol Health Care Res II* 1992;4:827A.
9. O'Hanlon JF, Ramaekers JG. Antihistamine effects on actual driving performance in a standard test: A summary of Dutch experience, 1989–1994. *Allergy* 1995;50(3):234–242.
10. Ray WA, Thapa PB, Shorr RI. Medications and the older driver. *Clin Geriatr Med* 1993;9(2):413–438.
11. Ray WA, Fought RL, Decker MD. Psychoactive drugs and the risk of injurious motor vehicle crashes in elderly patients. *Am J Epidemiol* 1992;136:873–883.
12. Skegg DCG, Richards SM, Doll R. Minor tranquilisers and road accidents. *Br Med J* 1979;1:917–919.
13. U.S. Department of Transportation, Federal Highway Administration. *Conference on Psychiatric Disorders and Commercial Drivers.* Publication No. FHWA-MC-91-006. Washington: U.S. DOT, Federal Highway Administration, Office of Motor Carriers, 1991.

14. Driver and Vehicle Licensing Agency. At-a-Glance Guide to the Current Medical Standards of Fitness to Drive. Swansea, England: Drivers Medical Unit, DVLA. *http://www.dvla.gov.uk/at_a_glance/ content.htm.* Accessed Dec. 9, 2002.

15. Grabe HJ, Wolf T, Grätz S, Laux G. The influence of polypharmacological antidepressive treatment on central nervous information processing of depressed patients: Implications for fitness to drive. *Neuropsychobiology* 1998;37:200–204.

16. Canadian Medical Association. Physicians' Guide to Driver Examination. *http://www.cma.ca/cma/common/displayPage.do?pageId=/ staticContent/HTML/publications/catalog/driversguide/index.htm.* Accessed Dec. 9, 2002.

17. Drugs for depression and anxiety. *Med Lett Drugs Ther* 2002;44(1140):83.

18. Barkley RA, Guevremont DC, Anastopoulos AD, et al. Driving-related risks and outcomes of attention deficit hyperactivity disorder in adolescents and young adults: A 3- to 5-year follow-up survey. *Pediatrics* 1993;92(2):212–218.

19. Nada-Raja S, Langley JD, McGee R, et al. Inattentive and hyperactive behaviors and driving offenses in adolescence. *J Am Acad Child Adolesc Psychol* 1997;36:515–522.

20. Barkley RA, Murphy KR, Depaul GJ, Bush T. Driving in young adults with attention deficit hyperactivity disorder: Knowledge, performance, adverse outcomes, and the role of executive functioning. *J Int Neuropsychol Soc* 2002;8:655–672.

21. Myers JK, Weissman MM, Tischler GE, et al. Six-month prevalence of psychiatric disorders in three communities. *Arch Gen Psychiatry* 1984;41:959–970.

22. Grabe HJ, Wolf T, Gratz S, Laux G. The influence of polyphar-macological antidepressive treatment on central nervous information processing of depressed patients: Implications for fitness to drive. *Neuropsychobiology* 1998;37(4):200–204.

23. Fong G, Frost D, Stansfeld S. Road rage: A psychiatric phenomenon? *Soc Psychiatry Psychiatr Epidemiol* 2001;36:277–286.

24. Grabe HJ, Wolf T, Grätz S, Laux G. The influence of clozapine and typical neuroleptics on information processing of the central nervous system under clinical conditions in schizophrenic disorders: Implications for fitness to drive. *Neuropsychobiology* 1999;40:196–201.

10

Renal Disease

NATALIE P. HARTENBAUM, MD, MPH

While there is no regulation that directly addresses drivers with renal disease, a number do so indirectly, including the cardiac, hypertension, respiratory, psychiatric, and neurologic standards. In evaluating the fitness of a commercial driver with renal disease, it is important not only to consider the renal disease itself but also to assess other coexisting medical conditions. Drivers with diabetes, hypertension, or heart disease may be at higher risk of complications and sudden impairment than drivers with renal disease alone.

Diabetic nephropathy, which may be due to either insulin-dependent or non–insulin-dependent diabetes, is the leading cause of end-stage renal disease in the United States and most industrialized countries [1]. Renal failure can result in a number of physiologic and clinical abnormalities. The average yearly mortality in patients on dialysis is about 25 percent, mostly from cardiovascular causes [2]. The first step in the evaluation must be to assess the degree of renal impairment. Results from laboratory studies, including determinations of electrolyte levels, blood urea nitrogen level, creatinine level, and creatinine clearance, should be reviewed, as should the degree of proteinuria, if present. There is some evidence that older drivers with proteinuria have an increased risk of motor vehicle accidents [3].

More than 50 percent of patients undergoing dialysis continue to have hypertension [4]. The advisory criteria for hypertension suggest that as part of the evaluation of the severity of hypertension, renal function should be evaluated. The criteria further suggest that individuals with a creatinine level > 2.5 mg/dL not be certified to drive commercial vehicles in interstate commerce.

Cardiovascular disease is the cause of death in up to 40 percent of patients with end-stage renal disease [5]. This increase continues even after renal transplantation. There is a five times increased relative risk of death from myocardial infarction in patients on any type of renal replacement therapy compared with the general population [6]. Aside from the high risk of myocardial ischemia, a number of other clinical cardiac abnormalities may be found in these patients. Renal failure may result in fluid overload, leading to congestive heart failure and pulmonary edema. Both of these may be controlled through dialysis and usually resolve after renal transplantation. Pericarditis and cardiomyopathy also may be seen. In one study, left ventricular cavity volume and left ventricular mass were predictive of death from cardiovascular causes in patients with renal failure [7].

Anemia also is common in patients with end-stage renal disease. The degree of anemia should be evaluated in a commercial driver because it leads to many of the problems seen in these patients. Such problems include fatigue and exercise intolerance as well as cardiac ischemia through a decreased amount of oxygen delivered to the cardiac tissue. Recombinant human erythropoietin improves both quality of life and overall function [8].

A mixed sensory and motor neuropathy, often more severe in the legs than in the arms, is common in patients with uremia. This often will respond to dialysis [9]. Diabetic neuropathy may be superimposed on the uremic neuropathy and will not improve with dialysis.

Abnormalities that may be seen in individuals with renal failure and affect their ability to concentrate include fatigue, impaired mentation, sleep disorders, restless legs syndrome (resulting in sleep disturbance), and peripheral neuropathies. In more severe cases, seizures or coma may occur if the uremia is not treated properly.

Two types of dialysis are used—hemodialysis or peritoneal dialysis. Hemodialysis is more common and usually requires 9 to 12 hours of treatment per week, often divided into three sessions per week. Frequently, an artificial shunt is used, and thus the incidence of infection or sepsis is high. The significant interruption in normal activities of daily living and altered body image may lead to depression. During dialysis, fluxes in osmolality and electrolytes may lead to a dialysis disequilibrium syndrome or arrhythmias. Hypotension is common. Electrolyte disturbances also may result in muscle cramps. The development of dialysis dementia is another concern.

Heparin is used during the dialysis procedure and may lead to subdural hematoma and retroperitoneal, gastrointestinal, pericardial, or pleural hemorrhage. Long-term dialysis patients have increased mortality due to myocardial infarction and cerebrovascular accidents, both serious concerns in a commercial driver. Dialysis is best performed in a consistent setting, a difficulty for many long-haul truckers. Arranging dialysis in different locations over the course of several weeks may be a logistical impossibility. A reliable schedule is also required and may present difficulty. Commercial drivers whose routes are solely local, short haul, or intermittent may be able to coordinate their work schedule around their dialysis schedule. Medical examiners, however, are unable to restrict drivers to operating only under these conditions. If it is determined that such a driver should be medically qualified, only short-term certification to monitor the disease process and work routine should be considered.

The other main method of dialysis is continuous ambulatory peritoneal dialysis (CAPD). For this method, patients instill dialysate fluid into the peritoneal cavity, seal the catheter, and continue with normal activities. The fluid is removed and replaced every 4 to 6 hours. A cyclic dialysate delivery device allows continuous exchange at night. Advantages over hemodialysis include the more gradual shifts in fluid and electrolyte levels and the avoidance of heparinization. Longer treatment times may be a disadvantage to some patients. Complications include catheter infection, peritonitis, and moderate protein loss. Since CAPD is performed by the patient, the requirement for compliance to avoid infection or other complications is significant.

Patients who undergo renal transplantation often will return to a near-normal lifestyle. One of the greatest risks for these individuals is transplant rejection. Such patients should be able to obtain care in the event of infection or rejection in a reasonable period of time. The risk of rejection is highest in the first year after transplantation. For a commercial driver, one concern should be the potential side effects of the medication in addition to its immunosuppressive effects. Steroids at higher doses can cause confusion, and cyclosporine can lead to tremor. As with all medication use in commercial drivers, it is important for examiners to be in contact with the treating physician to obtain an understanding of the medication and any potential interference with the safe operation of a vehicle.

Even with treatment, only about 10 to 20 percent of chronic renal failure patients are totally rehabilitated by dialysis, and another 30 to 40 percent of nondiabetic patients are returned to a functional level. Mean mortality for all end-stage renal disease patients is approximately 18 percent per year. In those younger than age 45 with no complicating medical problems, mortality with treatment falls below 5 percent per year.

As examiners under the Federal program, we are unable to limit geographic range or duration of driving or impose other restrictions. Patients often complain of weakness or fatigue the day after they are dialyzed, and the examiner will be unable to control for this.

Other Standards and Guidelines

In general, guidelines from other transportation modes and countries advise against certifying individuals on dialysis or after renal transplantation for performing safety-sensitive operations unless their condition is fully stabilized and thoroughly evaluated. The Federal Aviation Administration considers renal dialysis as a cause for denial of licensure except under limited circumstances. Australia's guidelines for commercial drivers consider a person with end-stage renal disease as not qualified unless an approved specialist supports a conditional license [10]. The Canadian Medical Association (CMA) advises that drivers on intermittent dialysis or continuous peritoneal dialysis can drive if they are otherwise in good health and that they can drive any class of vehicle but should be able to arrange for treatment and anticipate possible delays [11]. The CMA explains that the commercial driver must be under the care of a nephrologist or internist and must have an annual review. There also would have to be close cooperation among patient, physician, and licensing agency. For the commercial driver on dialysis or after transplantation, close follow-up and a requirement that the treating physician notify the licensing agency if the condition changes are also recommended.

In the United Kingdom, the Driver and Vehicle Licensing Agency's [12] medical group assesses commercial drivers on peritoneal or hemodialysis on an individual basis.

Conclusion

End-stage renal disease has the potential to cause sudden incapacitation in a commercial driver by a number of mechanisms. It is important to evaluate not only the degree and stability of renal impairment but also the presence and status of any coexisting diseases. Information from all treating physicians should be reviewed, and arrangements should be made with the primary treating physician that commercial driving status be reviewed with significant changes in medical stability. A recent accident with multiple fatalities involved a driver who was medically qualified and 2 months later began renal dialysis. No evaluation of the individual's ability to perform commercial driver functions occurred at that time or after long-term absences to stabilize his disease. Final determination of the actual cause of the accident is still pending, but the contribution of his medical condition has many people discussing the inadequacy of the current medical certification system.

References

1. Nuhad I, Becker B, Strzelczyk P, Ritz E. Renal disease and hypertension in non-insulin-dependent diabetes mellitus. *Kidney Int* 1999;55:1–28.
2. Renal Data System. *USRDS 1997 Annual Data Report.* Bethesda, MD: National Institute of Diabetes and Digestive and Kidney Disease, 1997.
3. Stewart RB, Moore MT, Marks RG, et al. *Driving Cessation and Accidents in the Elderly: An Analysis of Symptoms, Diseases, Cognitive Dysfunction and Medications.* Washington: AAA Foundation for Traffic Safety, 1993.
4. Pastan S, Bailey J. Medical progress: Dialysis therapy. *N Engl J Med* 1998;338:1428–1437.
5. Walker R. Recent advances: General management of end-stage renal disease. *Br Med J* 1997;315:1429–1432.
6. Raine AEG, MacMahon SH, Selwood NH, et al. Mortality from myocardial infarction in patients on renal replacement therapy in the UK. *Nephrol Dial Transplant* 1991;6:902–910.
7. Foley RN, Parfrey PS, Harnett JD, et al. The prognostic importance of left ventricular geometry in uremic cardiomyopathy. *J Am Soc Nephrol* 1995;5:2024–2031.
8. Canadian Erythropoietin Study Group. Association between recombinant human erythropoietin and quality of life and exercise capacity of patients requiring haemodialysis. *Br Med J* 1990;300:573–578.
9. Onyekachi I. Current concepts: Care of patients undergoing hemodialysis. *N Engl J Med* 1998;339:1054–1062.
10. Australasian Faculty of Occupational Medicine. *Medical Examinations of Commercial Vehicle Drivers.* Prepared for the National Road Transport Commission and the Federal Office of Road Safety, Sydney, Australia, 1997. *http://www.nrtc.gov.au/publications/medstand.asp?lo=public.* Assessed Oct. 14, 2002.
11. Canadian Medical Association. *Physicians' Guide to Driver Examination,* 6th ed. Ottawa, Canada: CMA, 2000.
12. Driver and Vehicle Licensing Agency. At-a-Glance Guide to the Current Medical Standards of Fitness to Drive. Swansea, England: Drivers Medical Unit, DVLA, Last updated August 2002. *http://www.dvla.gov.uk/at_a_glance/content.htm.* Assessed Oct. 14, 2002.

11

Substance Abuse and Medication Use

Natalie P. Hartenbaum, MD, MPH

Few areas have undergone as many changes in the commercial driver medical certification area as medication use and abuse and substance abuse. Two of the thirteen medical standards have addressed substance abuse since implementation of the standards. For a period of time, drug and alcohol testing were almost part of the periodic examination process. The new examination reporting form emphasizes the importance of reviewing the use of both prescription and nonprescription medications and the potential impact on safety that these medications may have. Included on the form is a statement that the medical examiner must review and discuss with the driver the "potential hazards including over-the-counter medications, while driving."

Drug and alcohol testing by the U.S. Department of Transportation (DOT) were begun in 1989 and 1994, respectively, after several high-profile accidents in which these substances were implicated as the probable cause. Although the Medical Review Officer (MRO) is responsible for determining whether there is a legitimate medical explanation for a laboratory non–negative test result, the examiner is required to determine whether the driver is using any substance that may pose a fitness-for-duty concern. There are several situations in which the MRO's and the examiner's paths may cross, and it is recognized that at times physicians may seem to serve as both MRO and examiner simultaneously. In practice, the two roles should be separate and the physician should "take off one hat and put on the other" when acting as either examiner or MRO.

This chapter does not discuss the MRO process except where it overlaps with a fitness-for-duty determination. Additional information on 49 CFR Part 40 or 49 CFR 382, the DOT or Federal Motor Carrier Safety Administration (FMCSA) regulations, respectively, can be found through the DOT (*http://www.dot.gov*) or FMCSA (*http://*

www.fmcsa.dot.gov) Internet sites. Another excellent resource is the DOT's Office of Drug and Alcohol Policy Compliance (*http://www.dot.gov/ost/dapc/*).

The Federal Motor Safety Regulations that address substance abuse and alcohol misuse [49 CFR 391.41(b)] state that a person is physically qualified to drive a commercial motor vehicle (CMV) if that person

"(12)(i) Does not use a controlled substance identified in 21 CFR 1308.11 Schedule I, an amphetamine, a narcotic, or any other habit-forming drug.

(ii) Exception. A driver may use such a substance or drug, if the substance or drug is prescribed by a licensed medical practitioner who:

(A) Is familiar with the driver's medical history and assigned duties; and

(B) Has advised the driver that the prescribed substance or drug will not adversely affect the driver's ability to safely operate a commercial motor vehicle; and

(13) Has no current clinical diagnosis of alcoholism."

Drivers who test positive under the DOT controlled substance testing regulations [1] are disqualified from operating CMVs. A recent change in the regulations will also lead to disqualification of drivers convicted of a drug- or alcohol-related offense while operating a passenger vehicle.

Advisory Criteria and Regulatory Guidance

The advisory criteria [2] for this part further explain the exception permitting drivers who are using a Schedule I controlled substance, an amphetamine, a narcotic, or any other habit-forming drug. Examiners must determine whether the medication or the medical condition it is treating may impair the driver's safe operation of the CMV. It is advised that a written statement be obtained from the prescribing provider. The controlled substances referenced in 49 CFR 391(b)12 (i) are found in 21 CFR 1308.11 (Figure 11-1). Methadone is specifically mentioned in the advisory criteria as well as in the Regulatory Guidance [3] as not being subject to this exception, and commercial drivers on methadone should be found medically unqualified.

Figure 11-1. Title 21—Food and Drugs. Section 1308.11 Schedule I.

TITLE 21—FOOD AND DRUGS
CHAPTER II—DRUG ENFORCEMENT ADMINISTRATION,
DEPARTMENT OF JUSTICE
PART 1308—SCHEDULES OF CONTROLLED SUBSTANCES—
 Table of Contents
Sec. 1308.11 Schedule I.

 (a) Schedule I shall consist of the drugs and other substances, by whatever official name, common or usual name, chemical name, or brand name designated, listed in this section. Each drug or substance has been assigned the DEA Controlled Substances Code Number set forth opposite it.

 (b) Opiates. Unless specifically excepted or unless listed in another schedule, any of the following opiates, including their isomers, esters, ethers, salts, and salts of isomers, esters and ethers, whenever the existence of such isomers, esters, ethers and salts is possible within the specific chemical designation (for purposes of paragraph (b)(34) only, the term isomer includes the optical and geometric isomers):

 (1) Acetyl-alpha-methylfentanyl (N-[1-(1-methyl-2-phenethyl)-4-piperidinyl]-N-phenylacetamide) 9815
 (2) Acetylmethadol 9601
 (3) Allylprodine 9602
 (4) Alphacetylmethadol (except levo-alphacetylmethadol also known as levo-alpha-acetylmethadol, levomethadyl acetate, or LAAM) 9603
 (5) Alphameprodine 9604
 (6) Alphamethadol 9605
 (7) Alpha-methylfentanyl (N-[1-(alpha-methyl-beta-phenyl)ethyl-4-piperidyl] propionanilide); 1-(1-methyl-2-phenylethyl)-4-(N-propanilido) piperidine) 9814
 (8) Alpha-methylthiofentanyl (N-[1-methyl-2-(2-thienyl)ethyl-4-piperidinyl]-N-phenylpropanamide) 9832
 (9) Benzethidine 9606
 (10) Betacetylmethadol 9607
 (11) Beta-hydroxyfentanyl (N-[1-(2-hydroxy-2-phenethyl)-4-piperidinyl]-N-phenylpropanamide) 9830
 (12) Beta-hydroxy-3-methylfentanyl (other name: N-[1-(2-hydroxy-2- phenethyl)-3-methyl-4-piperidinyl]-N-phenylpropanamide) 9831
 (13) Betameprodine 9608
 (14) Betamethadol 9609
 (15) Betaprodine 9611
 (16) Clonitazene 9612
 (17) Dextromoramide 9613
 (18) Diampromide 9615
 (19) Diethylthiambutene 9616
 (20) Difenoxin 9168

Figure 11-1. (*continued*)

(c) Opium derivatives. Unless specifically excepted or unless listed in another schedule, any of the following opium derivatives, its salts, isomers, and salts of isomers whenever the existence of such salts, isomers, and salts of isomers is possible within the specific chemical designation:

(*continued*)

Figure 11-1. (*continued*)

(d) Hallucinogenic substances. Unless specifically excepted or unless listed in another schedule, any material, compound, mixture, or preparation, which contains any quantity of the following hallucinogenic substances, or which contains any of its salts, isomers, and salts of isomers whenever the existence of such salts, isomers, and salts of isomers is possible within the specific chemical designation (for purposes of this paragraph only, the term "isomer" includes the optical, position and geometric isomers):

(1) Alpha-ethyltryptamine..................................... 7249
       Some trade or other names: etryptamine; Monase; [alpha]-ethyl-1H-indole-3-ethanamine; 3-(2-aminobutyl) indole; [alpha]-ET; and AET.
(2) 4-bromo-2,5-dimethoxy-amphetamine........................... 7391
       Some trade or other names: 4-bromo-2,5-dimethoxy-[alpha]-methylphenethylamine; 4-bromo-2,5-DMA.
(3) 4-bromo-2,5-dimethoxyphenethylamine......................... 7392
       Some trade or other names: 2-(4-bromo-2,5-dimethoxyphenyl)-1-aminoethane; alpha-desmethyl DOB; 2C-B, Nexus.
(4) 2,5-dimethoxyamphetamine.................................... 7396
       Some trade or other names: 2,5-dimethoxy-[alpha]-methylphenethylamine; 2,5-DMA.
(5) 2,5-dimethoxy-4-ethylamphetamine........................... 7399
       Some trade or other names: DOET.

Figure 11-1. (*continued*)

(*continued*)

Figure 11-1. (*continued*)

Synthetic equivalents of the substances contained in the plant,
or in the resinous extractives of Cannabis, sp. and/or synthetic
substances, derivatives, and their isomers with similar chemical
structure and pharmacological activity such as the following:
[Delta]1 cis or trans tetrahydrocannabinol, and their optical isomers
[Delta]6 cis or trans tetrahydrocannabinol, and their optical isomers
[Delta]3,4 cis or trans tetrahydrocannabinol, and its optical isomers
(Since nomenclature of these substances is not internationally
standardized, compounds of these structures, regardless of
numerical designation of atomic positions covered.)
Some trade or other names: N-ethyl-1-phenylcyclohexylamine,
(1- phenylcyclohexyl)ethylamine, N-(1-phenylcyclohexyl)
ethylamine, cyclohexamine, PCE.
Some trade or other names: 1-(1-phenylcyclohexyl)-pyrrolidine,
PCPy, PHP.
Some trade or other names: 1-[1-(2-thienyl)-cyclohexyl]-
piperidine, 2-thienylanalog of phencyclidine, TPCP, TCP.
Some other names: TCPy.

(e) Depressants. Unless specifically excepted or unless listed in another
schedule, any material, compound, mixture, or preparation which contains
any quantity of the following substances having a depressant effect on the
central nervous system, including its salts, isomers, and salts of isomers
whenever the existence of such salts, isomers, and salts of isomers is possible
within the specific chemical designation:

(1) gamma-hydroxybutyric acid (some other names include GHB;
    gamma-hydroxybutyrate; 4-hydroxybutyrate; 4-hydroxybutanoic
    acid; sodium oxybate; sodium oxybutyrate) 2010
(2) Mecloqualone 2572
(3) Methaqualone 2565

(f) Stimulants. Unless specifically excepted or unless listed in another
schedule, any material, compound, mixture, or preparation which contains
any quantity of the following substances having a stimulant effect on the
central nervous system, including its salts, isomers, and salts of isomers:

Figure 11-1. (*continued*)

(1) Aminorex (Some other names: aminoxaphen; 2-amino-5-phenyl-2-oxazoline; or 4,5-dihydro-5-phenly-2-oxazolamine). 1585
(2) Cathinone 1235
  Some trade or other names: 2-amino-1-phenyl-1-propanone,
  alpha-aminopropiophenone, 2-aminopropiophenone, and
  norephedrone
(3) Fenethylline 1503
(4) Methcathinone (Some other names: 2-(methylamino)-
  propiophenone; alpha-(methylamino)propiophenone; 2
  -(methylamino)-1-phenylpropan-1-one; alpha-N-
  methylaminopropiophenone; monomethylpropion; ephedrone;
  N-methylcathinone; methylcathinone; AL-464; AL-422; AL-463
  and UR1432), its salts, optical isomers and salts of optical
  isomers) 1237
(5) ([plusmn])cis-4-methylaminorex (([plusmn])cis-4,5-dihydro-
  4-methyl-5-phenyl-2-oxazolamine) 1590
(6) N-ethylamphetamine 1475
(7) N,N-dimethylamphetamine (also known as N,N-alpha-
  trimethyl-benzene-ethanamine; N,N-alpha-trimethyl-
  phenethylamine) 1480

(g) Temporary listing of substances subject to emergency scheduling. Any material, compound, mixture, or preparation which contains any quantity of the following substances:

(1) N-[1-benzyl-4-piperidyl]-N-phenylpropanamide (benzylfentanyl),
  its optical isomers, salts, and salts of isomers 9818
(2) N-[1-(2-thienyl)methyl-4-piperidyl]-N-phenylpropanamide
  (thenylfentanyl), its optical isolers, salts, and salts of isomers 9834

An examiner may determine use through interview, available history, or body fluid testing. If testing is done, it is not performed as DOT-required testing (do not use a Federal form), but any positive screening test should be confirmed. The advisory criteria indicate that if the driver is found to be medically unqualified owing to prohibited drug use, he or she can only return once a second examination finds that the driver is no longer using that substance. An evaluation by a substance abuse professional, completion of a drug rehabilitation program, and a negative drug test result may be required of a driver who was not qualified because of substance use. If a driver is found not to be medically qualified because of a regulated test which is MRO positive, a return to duty would have to include all of the components required by the DOT and FMCSA drug testing regulations. The examiner may also certify the driver for less than 2 years if there is a concern that there may be a recurrence of impairing or illegal substance use. As with all of the updated advisory criteria, the examiner is referred to the Conference Reports, for this standard, the Neurologic [4] and Psychiatric [5] reports.

For drivers found not to be medically qualified because of alcohol use, it is explained that "current clinical diagnosis" refers to a "current alcoholic illness or those instances where the individual's physical condition has not fully stabilized." This would seem not to include individuals who are abstinent and have no other alcohol-related medical conditions but who may be considered recovering alcoholics. Individuals who have physical signs of or provide a history consistent with alcohol problems should be referred to a specialist and, after evaluation and/or treatment, if indicated, should then be medically certified.

There was a great deal of confusion when DOT-mandated controlled substance testing was first implemented. At the time, the form included options that would allow the examiner to indicate whether the testing was performed "in accordance with subpart H" and whether controlled testing was performed as part of the medical examination. This was important because if the testing was part of the examination, then the examiner should not sign the medical certificate until the drug test results are reviewed and an MRO-negative report is obtained. The drug testing and examination are now totally separate procedures, and the only time they might ordinarily be performed at the same office visit would be in the preplacement setting [6]. The drug test, but not the examination, can be done prior to an offer of employment. The Regulatory Guidance explains that when a driver presents for both the drug test and the examination, the examination is completed first; if the driver meets the medical criteria, the medical certificate should be prepared. The collection for controlled substance testing is then performed. It is the motor carrier's responsibility to ensure that a verified negative test from the MRO has been obtained prior to having the driver operate CMVs. The examiner should not hold the card pending the controlled substance test result.

The Regulatory Guidance also addresses whether a driver who tests positive for alcohol or a controlled substance under part 382 needs a new medical examination. Provided that the driver was evaluated by a substance abuse professional (SAP) who did not determine that the driver had a current clinical diagnosis of alcoholism, a new examination is not required. If it is determined that the driver has a diagnosis of alcoholism, then the driver is not qualified. Again, the motor carrier is responsible for ensuring that the driver is medically qualified. This may be done through the SAP, but some carriers may choose to have the driver obtain a new medical certificate.

There are instances in which an examiner is performing an examination on a driver for one company and has previously provided MRO services on the same driver for another company. The Regulatory Guidance explains that the examiner may decline to qualify the driver if "the medical examiner determines, based on other evidence besides the drug test, including, but not limited to, knowledge of the prior positive test result, that the driver continues to use prohibited drugs 49 CFR 391.43." Many examiners in this situation will require information from a SAP prior to completing the certificate. The carrier is responsible for querying past employers about previous positive tests, and now must also ask about tests performed as preemployment. Any recommendation from the SAP regarding follow-up testing should also follow that driver to a new employer.

An examiner may have knowledge that could impact a fitness determination obtained while acting as an MRO for a different carrier. This may occur when a driver has a laboratory-positive test but the MRO determines that there is a legitimate medical explanation for the test result yet has concerns about whether that substance may impair the driver. The new 49 CFR Part 40 (49 CFR Part 40.327) directs the MRO to report information obtained in the verification process to an employer, physician, or other health care provider "responsible for determining the medical qualification of the employee under an applicable DOT agency safety regulation." This can be done without employee consent if it is determined that the information may result in the individual being medically unqualified because of a safety risk. Initially this was believed to prohibit reporting of the safety concern to a medical examiner for an employer other than the one for whom the test was performed. The September 2001 Q & A issued by the Office of Drug and Alcohol Policy Compliance [7] explains that if the MRO knew the identity of the physician responsible for determining whether the driver was physically qualified under FMCSA regulations for another employer, they could provide the information to that examiner. If the MRO serves as the medical examiner for another company, he or she can "take off" the MRO hat and essentially notify himself or herself as examiner for the other company that there may be a safety concern and that the driver would need to be evaluated [8].

The MRO may also report a negative test conducted under DOT regulations when the employee is unable to provide a urine specimen in the preplacement, return-to-duty, or follow-up situation (49 CFR Part 40.195). If the MRO determines that a permanent or long-term, preexisting condition prevents the individual from providing a sufficient urine specimen, he or she can conduct an examination, or have an examination conducted by a physician acceptable to the MRO, to determine whether there is clinical evidence of illicit drug use. Although the conditions may be met to report the test result as negative, the medical condition resulting in this inability to provide a urine specimen may cause the driver *not* to meet the medical criteria.

When state laws were passed legalizing medicinal marijuana, there were questions on how this would affect Federal drug testing policies. Federico Peña, then secretary of the U.S. DOT, stated on December 12, 1996, that "any safety-sensitive transportation worker—such as a pilot, railroad engineer, or bus driver—who tests positive under our program may not use Proposition 215 or Proposition 200 as an excuse or defense" [9]. He also explained that the MRO should not find that the presence of these substances, even *with* the report of a recommendation of a physician, is due to a legitimate medical use. Use of these substances is not consistent with Federally approved use.

Additional Considerations

Controlled Substances and Alcohol

In 2000, an estimated 14 million Americans were current (used in month preceding interview) illicit drug users [10]. Marijuana was the most commonly used—76% of illicit drug users. An estimated 7 million people reported driving under the influence of controlled substances, and most of those (77 percent) had also driven under the influence of alcohol.

Federally mandated drug and alcohol testing has served as a deterrent in commercial drivers. In 1999, positive rates for controlled substances were 1.3% and for alcohol were 0.5% for levels greater than 0.02 and 0.2% for levels greater than 0.04. This is a significant decrease from 1995, when the rates were 2.8% for controlled substances and 0.14% for alcohol [11]. Although the violation rate during testing is low, Washington State's Operation Trucker Check found that truck drivers are still using substances that may impair safe operation of the CMV [12]. Voluntary testing, not falling into any of the Federal testing categories, for controlled substances was requested of 1079 drivers; 822 actually submitted urine specimens, 19 percent declined testing. Of the 822 drivers, 21 percent were positive for illicit, prescription, or over-the-counter medications; 9.5 percent were positive for central nervous system stimulants other than nicotine or caffeine; and 4.3 percent tested positive for cannabinoids.

A 2000 National Highway Traffic Safety Administration report found that 1 percent of drivers of large trucks involved in fatal accidents were intoxicated, significantly less than for operators of private vehicles [13].

Some of the physical findings an examiner may encounter in an individual with excessive alcohol use are spider angiomas, conjunctival injection, palmar erythema, tremor, hepatomegaly, gynecomastia, and testicular atrophy. Slurred speech, unsteady gait, lack of attention to personal hygiene, tremor, and memory deficits may be observed when controlled substances or alcohol is abused.

Several tools can be used to screen for possible alcohol misuse [14]. One is the CAGE questionnaire. Positive responses to two or more of the following questions may indicate that further evaluation may be warranted:

1. Have you ever felt you should Cut down on your drinking?
2. Have people Annoyed you by criticizing your drinking?
3. Have you ever felt bad or Guilty about your drinking?
4. Have you ever had a drink first thing in the morning to steady your nerves or get rid of a hangover (Eye-opener)?

Others tools include the TWEAK scale and the Alcohol Use Disorders Identification Test (AUDIT) (Figure 11-2).

Findings that might lead an examiner to consider a diagnosis of drug use include needle tracks, a perforated nasal septum, a long curved fifth fingernail, dilated pupils (e.g., amphetamine, barbiturate, cocaine, marijuana, or lysergic acid diethylamide [LSD] use or opiate withdrawal), or constricted pupils (e.g., opiate use).

Prescription and Over-the-Counter Medications

Even more challenging for the medical examiner than determining whether the driver who drinks a few beers at night presents a danger on the road is whether a medication may impair. This includes both those prescribed by a health care professional and those purchased over the counter. The examiner is required to review with the driver any medications he or she may be taking and to discuss potential hazards. This might include advising drivers to read all package inserts, with special attention to precautions on driving or operating heavy machinery. A search of an electronic version of the *Physician's Desk Reference* found more than 700 medications with warnings similar to

Figure 11-2. TWEAK Scale

T   **Tolerance:** How many drinks does it take to make you feel high?

_____ No. of drinks

Score 2 points if 4 or more drinks for women, 6 or more for men

W   **Worry:** Have close friends or relatives worried or complained about your drinking in the past year? _____Yes _____No

Score 2 points for a positive "yes"

E   **Eye-Opener:** Do you sometimes have a drink in the morning when you first get up? _____Yes _____No

Score 1 point for a positive "yes"

A   **Amnesia (Blackouts):** Has a friend or family member ever told you about things you said or did while you were drinking that you could not remember? _____Yes _____No

Score 1 point for a positive "yes"

K(C) **Cut Down:** Do you sometimes feel the need to cut down on your drinking? _____Yes _____No

Score 1 point for a positive "yes"

A total score of 2 or more points indicates a likely drinking problem.

Alcohol Use Disorders Identification Test (AUDIT)

1. How often do you have a drink containing alcohol?
   _____ never (0)
   _____ monthly or less (1)
   _____ 2 to 4 times a month (2)
   _____ 2 to 3 times per week (3)
   _____ 4 or more times per week (4)

2. How many drinks containing alcohol do you have on a typical day when you are drinking?
   _____ not applicable (0)
   _____ 1 or 2 (0)
   _____ 3 or 4 (1)
   _____ 5 or 6 (2)
   _____ 7 to 9 (3)
   _____ 10 or more (4)

Figure 11-2. TWEAK Scale (*continued*)

3. How often do you have six or more drinks on one occasion?
   ____ not applicable/never (0)
   ____ less than monthly (1)
   ____ monthly (2)
   ____ weekly (3)
   ____ daily or almost daily (4)

4. How often during the past year have you found that you were not able to stop drinking once you had started?
   ____ not applicable/never (0)
   ____ less than monthly (1)
   ____ monthly (2)
   ____ weekly (3)
   ____ daily or almost daily (4)

5. How often during the past year have you failed to do what was normally expected from you because of drinking?
   ____ not applicable/never (0)
   ____ less than monthly (1)
   ____ monthly (2)
   ____ weekly (3)
   ____ daily or almost daily (4)

6. How often during the past year have you needed a first drink in the morning to get yourself going after a heavy drinking session?
   ____ not applicable/never (0)
   ____ less than monthly (1)
   ____ monthly (2)
   ____ weekly (3)
   ____ daily or almost daily (4)

7. How often during the past year have you had a feeling of guilt or remorse after drinking?
   ____ not applicable/never (0)
   ____ less than monthly (1)
   ____ monthly (2)
   ____ weekly (3)
   ____ daily or almost daily (4)

8. How often during the past year have you been unable to remember what happened the night before because you had been drinking?
   ____ not applicable/never (0)
   ____ less than monthly (1)
   ____ monthly (2)
   ____ weekly (3)
   ____ daily or almost daily (4)

(*continued*)

TWEAK **11-2.**   Tweak Scale (*continued*)

9. Have you or someone else been injured as a result of your drinking?
   ____ no (0)
   ____ yes, but not during the past year (2)
   ____ yes, during the past year (4)

10. Has a relative, friend, doctor, or other health worker been concerned about your drinking or suggested you cut down?
    ____ no (0)
    ____ yes, but not during the past year (2)
    ____ yes, during the past year (4)

____ TOTAL SCORE

Score by adding value in parenthes is next to selected response.

Sum ≥ 8 is considered positive for alcohol dependence or abuse.

"Use caution when driving a motor vehicle or operating machinery." Drivers should also be made aware that medications that list fatigue or sedation as side effects may not be safe to use while operating a CMV. In addition, it must be remembered, and the driver must be advised, that many over-the-counter medications contain alcohol and that side effects can be increased when certain medications are used with even small amounts of alcohol or other medications. The driver should not use these medications while driving until he or she or the physician is certain that there are no impairing side effects.

The advisory criteria instruct the examiner to discuss the effect a medication may have with the treating provider, but, unfortunately, the provider may not be aware or may be unable to assess the risk that a specific medication may have on safety. Similar to alcohol, an individual is often unable to determine whether he or she is impaired or the degree of impairment with a particular medication. By relying on subjective observations and whether drivers report them to a prescribing provider or the medical examiner is much like permitting individuals who have had several drinks to get behind the wheel because they do not believe they are impaired [15].

Medications in several classes, including the first-generation antihistamines, benzodiazepines, antidepressants, anxiolytics, narcotics, and some of the non-narcotic analgesics, have a high incidence of sedation as a side effect. Other side effects examiners must consider include dizziness, confusion, fatigue, seizures, headaches, and hypotension. Potential interactions among medications the driver might be using should also be evaluated. The examiner must educate drivers and providers on the well-documented risks of impairment with certain medications. Drivers and examiners should be encouraged to avoid use of these potentially impairing medications whenever possible by utilizing alternatives that do not have an undesirable side effect profile.

All medications must be used as approved by the Food and Drug Administration (FDA). Drivers should be instructed to always use medications as prescribed, not to increase the dose except under supervision, and to avoid driving until they know how the medication might affect them. They also should inform their health care provider of any and all medications, including herbal or alternative treatments, as side effects may be additive.

It is important that the examiner not only focus on the medication but on the underlying condition as well. Although the driver may be on a medication that has the potential to impair performance and the prescribing provider insists that the individual is not impaired, the underlying medical condition itself may interfere with safe operation of a CMV.

Over the years, the DOT has repeatedly reminded those in the transportation industries *"of potential threat to public safety caused by the on-duty use of some over-the-counter and prescription medication by persons performing some safety sensitive duties."* Employee training was recommended. As a result of studying more than 100 accidents in all modes of transportation that involved prescription or over-the-counter medications that could potentially impair the operator, the National Transportation Safety Board (NTSB) in 2000 recommended that the DOT develop a list of approved medications/classes of medications and forbid the use of medications not on the list for twice the dosage interval, except where individually assessed [16]. The NTSB recommends against relying on the individual's subjective assessment and reports of this assessment to the treating provider. The NTSB states in the 2000 safety recommendation that "vehicle operators using such medications might not always be in a position to judge the extent and effect of such impairment; a vehicle operator whose judgment is adversely affected by a medication may decide, inappropriately, that he or she is not impaired." Although the FDA has made labeling for over-the-counter medications more consistent, there is still concern that this may not be sufficient to adequately warn of potential hazards for those performing services in commercial transportation operations. There is no FDA requirement for labeling directed toward consumers for prescription medications. The package inserts, which may be provided to the individual, are directed at health care providers and are difficult to read and understand. Although labels may include precautions for driving and operating heavy machinery, this is based on subjective reports of sedation or drowsiness and not on specific tests that measure degree of impairment. Even if we can get drivers and health care providers to read the labels and consider the potential impairment, subjective reports of side effects do not correlate with actual performance decrements [17].

The NTSB and FDA held a joint public meeting in November 2001 to review the effects of medications on commercial operations. The main issues addressed in that meeting were

1. How to increase awareness of the public about the possible impairment caused by prescription and over-the-counter drug products

2. How to identify products that cause impairment

3. How to help the public avoid taking products that will cause impairment while driving

4. Whether relabeling those prescription and over-the-counter products helps the issue

The full transcript from that meeting is on the Internet at *http:// www.fda.gov/ohrms/dockets/dockets/01n0397/01n0397.htm*. Based on information from that meeting, the FDA plans to review and update labeling for several of the benzodiazepines and benzodiazepine-like hypnotics with intermediate and longer half-lives. They will also consider whether standard testing of the effect on driving performance should be required during drug development for potentially sedating drugs. The FDA did not indicate that it planned to review warnings on over-the-counter medication other than the new over-the-counter labeling. A public education campaign to give further attention to the need for consumers to comply with all labeling warnings, including those about drowsiness and driving, was mentioned as a consideration [18].

Several of the Conference Reports discussed medications. In the Cardiac report [19], it was suggested that antihypertensives with a higher incidence of drowsiness be avoided, including clonidine, methyldopa, guanabenz, reserpine, and prazosin. Medications that can cause postural hypotension should be used with caution. Headache medications that might cause sedation such as barbiturates, antihistamines, and analgesics were concerns for in the Neurology report [4].

Pulmonary conference [20] participants recommended against the use of antitussives and antihistamines for at least 12 hours prior to driving owing to their sedating side effects. This report noted that alternatives are available and "commercial drivers can and should avoid potentially sedating antihistamines." Since the Conference Reports, there have been studies [21] demonstrating impairment with the first-generation antihistamines. Others have demonstrated greater performance deficits in tests of divided attention, working memory, vigilance, and speed in subjects taking first-generation antihistamines compared with those on the newer, nonsedating agents and placebo [22]. This decrement in performance continued into the following day. When driving performance of sedating and nonsedating antihistamines were compared, the newer drugs were found to be less impairing, although none were unimpairing at one to two times the recommended doses [23]. In another study [24], driving simulator performance after a prototypic sedating antihistamine was worse than a illegal level of alcohol for driving. Importantly, in this study, subjective feelings of drowsiness did not correlate with impairment. Nonsedating antihistamines are an option, but they are currently available by prescription only. More than 60 percent of allergy sufferers had taken over-the-counter medications for their allergies, and in one survey, most indicated they were unaware of the difference between the sedating and nonsedating options [16].

The most extensive recommendations can be found in the Conference on Psychiatric Disorders and Commercial Drivers [5], in which all but the nonsedating anxiolytics were recommended to be disqualifying. It was also advised that only short-acting hypnotics be used, and for less than 2 weeks only. Drivers on antidepressants and antipsychotics were recommended to be referred to a psychiatrist for evaluation of both the condition and the medication side effects. Stimulants were also recommended to be disqualifying unless reviewed because although they can improve performance of simple tasks, they can impair performance of complex tasks.

In studies outside the Conference Reports, psychoactive medications such as the benzodiazepines [25–27] have been demonstrated to increase the risk of motor vehicle accidents. Alprazolam was found to cause serious driving impairment [28]. This study concluded that "alprazolam users must be warned not to drive an automobile or operate potentially dangerous machinery." In an economic assessment on the risk of a sleep medication, Menzin et al [29] estimated that the use of a driving-impairing sleep medication would result in about 503 excess accidents per 100,000 drivers during a 14-day period.

The examiner is in the difficult position of trying to determine whether a particular medication will interfere with a particular driver's performance. Many have utilized questionnaires or dialogue with the prescribing physician. Whenever possible, the driver should be on medications that do not impair. When new medications are started that carry the warning or precaution against driving or operating heavy machinery, the commercial driver should refrain from driving until he or she is aware of how the medication might affect his or her abilities.

Abuse of alcohol and controlled substances is a major problem for our society. As examining professionals, we hold an important role in protecting the driving public by certifying only those individuals who meet Federal Highway Administration criteria and who, to the best of our ability to detect, do not have a current problem with drugs or alcohol.

References

1. U.S. Department of Transportation, Office of the Secretary. Procedures for transportation workplace drug and alcohol testing programs: Final rule. *Fed Reg* 2000;65(Dec. 19):79461–79579.
2. Physical qualification of drivers: Medical examination—Final rule. *Fed Reg* 2000;65(Oct. 5):59363–59380.
3. Regulatory Guidance for the Federal Motor Carrier Safety Regulations, Department of Transportation, Federal Highway Administration, originally published April 4, 1997, available and updated at *http://www.fmcsa.dot.gov/rulesregs/fmcsr/fmcsrguide.htm*. Accessed Oct. 14, 2002.
4. U.S. Department of Transportation, Federal Highway Administration. *Conference on Neurological Disorders and Commercial Drivers*. Publication No. FHWA-MC-88-042. Washington: U.S. DOT, Federal Highway Administration, Office of Motor Carriers, 1988.
5. U.S. Department of Transportation, Federal Highway Administration. *Conference on Psychiatric Disorders and Commercial Drivers*. Publication No. FHWA-MC-91-006. Washington: U.S. DOT, Federal Highway Administration, Office of Motor Carriers, 1991.
6. Commercial driver's license program and controlled substances and alcohol use and testing—Conforming and technical amendments. *Fed Reg* 1997;62(July 11):37150–37153.
7. Office of Drug and Alcohol Policy Compliance. Questions and Answers, September 2001. *http://www.dot.gov/ost/dapc/*. Accessed Oct. 10, 2002.

8. Hartenbaum NP. MROs, medical examiner and positive drug tests. *CDME Review,* Fall 2002.

9. Peña F. *Statement on the Use of Proposition 200 and 215, December 12, 1996.* Washington: U.S. DOT, Office of the Assistant Secretary of Public Affairs, 1996.

10. *Summary of Findings From the 2000 National Household Survey on Drug Abuse.* Washington: Department of Health and Human Services, SAMHSA, Office of Applied Studies, September 2001.

11. U.S. Department of Transportation, Federal Motor Carrier Safety Administration. Controlled substances and alcohol testing management information system (MIS) statistical data: Notice. *Fed Reg* 2001;66(June 18):32862–32863.

12. Couper FJ, Pemberton M, Jarvis A, Hughes M, Logan BK. Prevalence of drug use in commercial tractor-trailer drivers. *J Forensic Sci* 2002;47(3):562–567.

13. *NHTSA Traffic Safety Facts 2000—Large Trucks.* DOT-HS-809-325. Washington: National Highway Traffic Safety Administration, 2001.

14. LoBuono C. Dealing with the alcohol controversy. *Patient Care* 2000;5:211–225.

15. Meltzer EO. Performance effects of antihistamines. *J Allergy Clin Immunol* 1990;86:613–619.

16. National Transportation Safety Board. Safety Recommendation. Public Meeting: Safety Recommendations to be Issued to the DOT and Other Agencies Concerning the Use of Medications by Vehicle Operators, January 5, 2000.

17. Kay GG, Quig ME. Impact of sedating antihistamines on safety and productivity. *Allergy Asthma Proc* 2001;22(5):281–283.

18. Correspondence from Steven Galson, MD, MPH, Deputy Director, Center for Drug Evaluation and Research, FDA, to Marion C. Blakey, Chairman, National Transportation Safety Board, June 21, 2002.

19. U.S. Department of Transportation, Federal Highway Administration. *Conference on Cardiac Disorders and Commercial Drivers.* Publication No. FHWA-MC-88-040. Washington: U.S. DOT, Federal Highway Administration, Office of Motor Carriers, 1987.

20. U.S. Department of Transportation, Federal Highway Administration. *Conference on Respiratory/Pulmonary Disorders and Commercial Drivers.* Publication No. FHWA-MC-91-004. Washington: U.S. DOT, Federal Highway Administration, Office of Motor Carriers, 1991.

21. Adelsberg BR. Sedation and performance issues in the treatment of allergic conditions. *Arch Intern Med* 1997;157:494–500.

22. Kay GG. The effects of antihistamines on cognition and

performance. *J Allergy Clin Immunol* 2000;105(6, pt 2)(suppl):S622–S627.

23. O'Hanlon JF, Ramaekers JG. Antihistamine effects on actual driving performance in a standard test: A summary of Dutch experience, 1989–94. *Allergy* 1995;50:234–242.

24. Weiler JM, Bloomfield JR, Woodworth GG, et al. Effects of fexofenadine, diphenhydramine, and alcohol on driving performance: A randomized, placebo-controlled trial in the Iowa Driving Simulator. *Ann Intern Med* 2000;132:354–363.

25. Barbone F, McMahon AD, Davey PG, et al. Association of road-traffic accidents with benzodiazepine use. *Lancet* 1998;352:1331–1336.

26. Hemmelgarn B, Suissa S, Huang A, Boivin JF, Pinard G. Benzodiazepine use and the risk of motor vehicle crash in the elderly. *JAMA* 1997;278:27–31.

27. Neutel CI. Risk of traffic injury after a prescription for a benzodiazepine. *Ann Epidemiol* 1995;5:239–244.

28. Verster JC, Volkerts ER, Verbaten MN. Effects of alprazolam on driving ability, memory functioning and psychomotor performance: a randomized, placebo-controlled study. *Neuropsychopharmacology* 2002;27(2):260–269.

29. Menzin J, Lang K, Levy P, Levy E. A general model of the effects of sleep medications on the risk and cost of motor vehicle accidents and its application to France. *Pharmacoeconomics* 2001;19:69–78.

Additional References

Fleming JAE. Pharmacological aspects of drowsiness, in Shapiro CM, Smith AM (eds.): *Forensic Aspects of Sleep.* Chicester, NY: John Wiley & Sons, 1997.

Grabe HJ, Wolf T, Gratz S, Laux G. The influence of clozapine and typical neuroleptics on information processing of the central nervous system under clinical conditions in schizophrenic disorders: Implications for fitness to drive. *Neuropsychobiology* 1999;40(4):196–201.

Grabe HJ, Wolf T, Gratz S, Laux G. The influence of polypharmacological antidepressive treatment on central nervous information processing of depressed patients: Implications for fitness to drive. *Neuropsychobiology* 1998;37(4):200–204.

Leveille SG, Buchner DM, Koepsell TD, McCloskey LW, Wolf ME, Wagner EH. Psychoactive medications and injurious motor vehicle collisions involving older drivers. *Epidemiology* 1994;5:591–598.

Logan BK, Case GA, Gordon AM. Carisoprodol, meprobamate, and driving impairment. *J Forensic Sci* 2000;45(3):619–623.

Ray WA, Purushottam BT, Shorr RI. Medications and the older driver. *Clin Geriatr Med* 1993;9:413–438.

Wylie KR, Thompson DJ, Wildgust HJ. Effects of depot neuroleptics on driving performance in chronic schizophrenic patients. *J Neurol Neurosurg Psychiatry* 1993;56(8):910–913.

III

Commercial Drivers' Health: Risks and Hazards

SAMUEL D. CAUGHRON, MD

In the twentieth century, many changes were made possible due to increased ease of transportation. Transportation of people and goods by animals and trains at the beginning of the century gave way to transportation by automobiles, commercial motor vehicles, and airplanes. In 1997, there were more than 7 million large trucks registered in the United States and more than 9.5 million commercial licenses, most held by people working as owner-drivers or for small companies [1].

A medical certification process has been instituted by most states and the Federal government to protect the public by ensuring that drivers are physically and mentally capable of driving safely. Belkic et al briefly state: "Professional driving is characterized by decision-making underload coupled with input high demand. It is primarily an avoidance activity performed under conditions of conflict, physical and mental constraint, time pressure and exposure to physically noxious agents (e.g., noise, glare, whole body vibration, lead, carbon monoxide, and other combustion products)" [2]. Simply put, driving alone is a high-stress occupation; however, today's commercial driver does much more than drive. The Professional Truck Driver Institute developed a set of skill standards, which includes the basic skills needed for tractor-trailer drivers [3] (Table III-1).

Today, driving a commercial motor vehicle may be considered a hazardous profession. In the 2001 Census of Fatal Occupational Injuries, truck drivers were found to have more workplace fatalities than any other individual occupation [4]. In 2001, truck drivers had a rate of 25.3 workplace fatalities per 100,000 employed. The incidence of injuries in those involved in trucking and courier services (except air) was 8.3 per 100 full-time workers in 2001 among private sector industries with 100,000 or more cases [5].

Of 41,471 fatal accidents in 1998 on the nation's highways, approximately 5375 involved large trucks, with occupants of the other vehicles consistently suffering more fatal injuries: 4572 vs 783 of the large truck occupants.

The Code of Federal Regulations, Title 49, Part 391.41, is the legal authority guiding medical evaluation of the commercial drivers. The recent 1998 Transportation Equity Act for the 21st Century amends part of this act as it pertains to waivers and exemptions, with changes in May of 2001. To evaluate and decide on driver fitness, the examiner must understand this law and its regulations, some basics about vehicle equipment and schedules, and the structure of the trucking industry. Examiners should also be aware of hazards and risks to the driver.

Table III-1. Skill standards for entry-level tractor-trailer drivers*

Read and Interpret Control Systems

Perform Vehicle Inspections

Exercise Basic Control

Execute Shifting

Back and Dock Tractor-Trailer

Couple Trailer

Uncouple Trailer

Perform Visual Search

Manage and Adjust Vehicle Speed

Manage and Adjust Vehicle Space Relations

Check and Maintain Vehicle Systems and Components

Diagnose and Report Malfunctions

Identify Potential Driving Hazards and Perform Emergency Maneuvers

Identify and Adjust to Difficult and Extreme Driving Conditions

Handle and Document Cargo

Deal with Accident Scenes and Reporting Procedures

Deal with Environmental Issues

Plan Trips/Make Appropriate Decisions

Use Effective Communication and Public Relations Skills

Manage Personal Resources/Deal with Life on the Road

Record and Maintain Hours of Service Requirements

---

*Tractor-trailer driver skills standards were developed through collaborative efforts of schools, truck drivers, trucking firms, and associations throughout the industry, building on data from the U.S. Department of Transportation and the Professional Truck Driver Institute [3].

Structure of the Trucking System

The trucking industry is composed of large commercial firms and governmental and private carriers. The Federal government has issued guidelines for commercial driver's license (CDL) medical examinations for the safety of the public. Many large companies and independent operations have established their own standards, policies, and procedures, which may go far beyond the regulated minimum. In contrast, many small and owner-driver operations have no policies beyond the Federal regulations. Therefore, it is important to determine what criteria are to be used in performing driver evaluations.

The commercial vehicle environment centers around the highway system. Access to food, fuel, communications, restrooms, bathing facilities, sleeping quarters, and so on, must be quick and easy to work into a driver's busy schedule. The myths of the "open road" are belied by the reality found in truck stops and interchanges around the United States. Fast food, high in fat and calories, fast motels near noisy highways, lack of exercise facilities, and tenuous spiritual and social environments make positive lifestyle choices difficult. In 1980, the trucking industry was deregulated, with salaries falling for commercial drivers from $52,000 the year before deregulation to $40,000 in 2001 [6].

Equipment

Under Federal requirements, a CDL is required to operate a motor vehicle involved in interstate commerce with a gross combination weight rating of 11,794 kilograms or more (26,001 pounds or more) inclusive of a towed unit with a gross vehicle weight rating of more than 4536 kilograms (10,000 pounds); or having a gross vehicle weight rating of 11,794 kilograms or more (26,001 pounds or more). Fully loaded, they can weigh about 80,000 pounds. A CDL is also required for the transportation of hazardous materials or for vehicles carrying sixteen or more passengers, including the driver. Some states use different weight cutoffs to define a commercial vehicle used in intrastate commerce.

Currently, there are more than 7 million commercial vehicles registered in the United States, as well as vehicles from Canada and Mexico plying our highways. Of these, 70 percent are straight (one-piece vehicles) and 30 percent are tractor-trailers [1]. Straight trucks have up to five axles and may appear as vans, flatbeds, or dump bodies. Their use is predominantly in local pick-up and delivery. Seventy percent of the nation's trucks are used mainly in local areas. Tractor-trailers consist of a power unit (tractor) and one to three trailers. They appear in many types, namely, "reefers" (refrigerators), dry van, flatbed, step-deck, tankers, livestock, grain, lowboy, specialized, etc. They may transport loads up to 50,000 pounds in long hauls. Many drivers are required to load and unload, and connect and disconnect their units, and this has important implications for physical requirements and potential injury. The large truck manufacturers have used technology to improve everything from instrumentation to sound and vibration control; however, many older vehicles still ply the roads. Cardiovascular measures suggest increased stress with driving the most demanding configuration (i.e., triple trailer A-dolly) [7].

Schedules

Typical work schedules vary [8]. On turnaround or short relay, a driver may drive 4 to 5 hours, leave the truck he or she has driven, and return in another vehicle. On long relays, a driver will drive up to 10 hours, take an 8-hour break, and then return. Straight-through hauling is often cross-country, with 10 hours of driving and 8-hour rest stops. In long-haul team driving, drivers share alternating 4-hour periods of driving, with 4-hour rest periods in the cab of the truck. Straight-haul and sleeper-haul drivers often are on the road for days to weeks. Laws in Canada and Mexico include different scheduling requirements. Scheduling issues have been sited as one of the primary stressors of commercial truckers [9]. A *New England Journal of Medicine* study noted that truck drivers typically slept 4.78 hours per day, 2 hours less than what drivers in the study determined was sufficient for job alertness [10]. Extended working time combined with greater load during a long-lasting trip may act to generate an internal desynchronization of circadian rhythms in long-haul tuck drivers [11]. Using self-reported data, the frequency of violation-inducing schedules was estimated during their ongoing movement for a sample of 498 long-distance drivers. Assuming average legal speed limits of 55 MPH, 26 percent of the drivers were found to have violation-inducing schedules. Solo drivers, drivers hauling refrigerated loads, regular route drivers, and those with longer current trip distances are the most likely to have such schedules. Also estimated were total weekly work hours. Assuming average attained traveling speeds of 50 MPH, the average driver drives 46 hours per week and works a total of 58 hours [12].

Hazards

Hazards facing the trucker may be mental, social, economic, or physical.

Mental Hazards

Mental factors and psycho-physiological hazards such as shifting work schedules and irregular work and rest cycles are complicated by difficulty with poor nutrition and unsatisfactory sleeping accommodations to create an extremely stressful environment [11]. Delays en route and traffic problems are quite common. Many drivers become anxious trying to meet schedules. The very act of driving can become quite monotonous, leading to fatigue [13]. The professional driver must deal with other drivers who may engage in unsafe, aggressive driving behavior in many different conditions [14]. Economic pressures involving owner-operators or those participating in small businesses add to the mental stressors. Sleep deprivation can be a major factor [10,15].The push to maximize service can create an environment in which drivers ignore legal mandates and push themselves to their physical limits [8,16]. Shift work, with frequent changing of sleep times, can disrupt circadian rhythms and create physiologic and emotional changes [17,18], and substances may be used to increase functioning, including tobacco, caffeine, and ephedrine, but both legal and illegal stimulants may be used. The monotony and frustration of driving can promote drowsiness and increase levels of aggression or apathy, both of which may increase the incidence of problems.

Socioeconomic Hazards

Social and economic factors also are present. With long-haul drivers away from home for up to several weeks, family pressures may become quite severe. Loneliness, exposure to illicit activities, drug use, and sexual situations are present. In one study of sexual activity among truck drivers in Florida, one third of the 71 men interviewed had frequent sexual intercourse on the road with multiple partners, but few ever used condoms. Commercial sex workers were their most frequent partners for on-the-road sex. The risk was compounded by occupational conditions, which motivated truckers to drive long hours, often using drugs to stay alert. Sex, alcohol, and drugs were perceived as quick, effective stress relievers during downtime on long, lonely trips. Despite their high-risk behaviors, truckers tended to consider themselves at low risk for human immunodeficiency virus (HIV) infection, and they expressed a number of misconceptions regarding HIV transmission. For example, many truckers did not associate HIV risk with heterosexual contact or think that condoms were effective in preventing HIV transmission. In addition, many truckers maintained strong homophobic and antigovernment opinions that reinforced their suspicion of safe-sex messages [19].

Most commercial vehicles not run by companies have brokers who arrange loads for the individual drivers. This can be a difficult situation, since individual owner-operators may have high levels of debt. The possible use of extortion to secure work or assist with loading or unloading may complicate a tenuous economic existence. The cost of a tractor may be more than $100,000, and incomes may be variable.

Physical Hazards

Physical factors affecting a driver can be internal or external to the vehicle and equipment. External factors such as time of day, degree of traffic, weather conditions, and road surfaces can vary considerably and alter alertness levels. Internal factors include driving position, ergonomic positioning of instruments, vibration, noise, heat, and physical conditioning.

Driving Position.   Driving position may vary dramatically. Some short-haul delivery vans may require a semi-standing position, whereas long-haul driving is predominantly sitting. Great strides have been made in adjusting the cab environment to the driver during the past 10 to 15 years [20]. Noise reduction, tinted windows, lumbar supports, adjustable seats, and antivibration devices are now available. Degenerative joint disease is more common in commercial drivers and occurs at an earlier age [21]. Measured changes in spinal pressure can be seen, and a documented increase in herniated disks is found among commercial drivers compared with others [22].

Vibration.   Vibration has been studied extensively. Measured in frequency, amplitude, velocity, and acceleration, it is the motion that forces a body out of a position or a state of equilibrium. Vibration may affect the cardiovascular, gastrointestinal, genitourinary, and musculoskeletal systems. In the bones, the increased rates of degenerative joint disease and disk disease mentioned previously are noted in truck drivers and may be a result of vibration. Disorders of the spine are common, with 50 percent of drivers reporting back pain. Magnusson et al's study in *Spine* suggested that a combination of long-term vibration exposure, heavy lifting, and frequent lifting carried the highest risk of low back pain [23].

Noise Hazards. The role of driver hearing in commercial vehicle operations has been studied recently. These studies suggest that "the overall mean broadband sound pressure level for truck-cab noise is very near the OSHA permissible exposure limit of 90 dBA for 8 hours. Truck-cab noise degrades communication in the truck to unacceptable levels under many conditions. Noise levels often mask both interior and exterior warning signals, thus impacting public safety" [24] Occupational Safety and Health Administration (OSHA) hearing conservation regulations apply to 8-hour time-weighted averages at 85 dB or greater. The National Institute of Occupational Safety and Health (NIOSH) currently sets a 90-dB limit, at which noise may adversely affect the temporary threshold value of a driver. Older cabs still found in the United States may have noise levels of up to 110 dB. Newer cabs with better sound conditioning have moderated this, but ambient highway noise may still cause noise levels in excess of 110 dB for short periods. Noise exposure can then produce a temporary hearing loss or temporary threshold shift. If repeated over prolonged periods, permanent hearing loss may occur. At noise levels as low as 70 dB, communication difficulties may occur (e.g., failure to hear emergency horns, sirens, etc.).

Heat Hazards. Heat gain caused by the sun shining through a truck cab's large windows, as well as climate variations, can create an adverse physical environment. Wet bulb-globe temperatures that take into account temperature, humidity, radiation, and wind speed can be measured. NIOSH considers above 79°F to be a hot environment [25]. Heat stress is moderated by perspiration, increased skin blood flow, heart rate increase, and hormonal changes. When heat is continuous, acclimatization can occur, but usually this takes 4 to 7 days. With wet bulb-globe temperatures over 88°F, however, acclimatization does not occur.

Air Quality Hazards. Drivers are exposed to fumes and high levels of pollutants in the highway environment. Engine emissions from their own and other engines create hydrocarbon exposure. Carbon monoxide exposure may also be present in confined or poorly ventilated spaces. There is some suggestion that there may be an increased incidence of cancers of the lung [26,27], emphysema, and other pulmonary diseases in commercial drivers [28]. Duration of exposure to diesel fumes seems to cause a trend of increased risk for lung cancer, accidents, cerebrovascular accidents, arteriosclerosis, and cirrhosis of the liver [29,30]. Cause and effect, however, have not been definitively established because concurrent conditions found in truck drivers, such as a high incidence of tobacco use, complicate the evaluation of respiratory diseases. Increased asthma and pulmonary-related conditions are also found in commercial drivers [31].

Visual Hazards. The very nature of the job creates a great stress on the ability of the brain to interpret visual stimuli [32]. Genetic factors regarding visual acuity and color-blindness are important to the safe operation of any motor vehicle. Commercial drivers constantly need to scan instruments, mirrors, and the road environment. Eye fatigue may be accentuated by vibration or exposure to glare and bright light. Poor weather conditions with decreased visibility encourage drivers to stretch their perceptions to the limit; this may increase the level of headaches. The aging driver may develop presbyopia, making visualization of the instruments more difficult.

Highway Maintenance

The entire highway system requires a tremendous amount of maintenance, from repair of potholes and clearing of snow to replacement of large segments of highway with accompanying bridges, overpasses, and so on. This work is time-consuming and expensive. Federal and state governments have the responsibility to attend to these issues; however, much of the repair has been deferred in difficult economic times. The driver, therefore, may need to negotiate a number of physical roadway challenges. While there is a trend for tractors to become bigger, with capacity for multiple trailers, there is not the same trend for the maintenance of road conditions necessary to support these vehicles. This dichotomy of bigger, heavier trucks with deteriorating road integrity increases driver stress. Poor road conditions can increase driver stress.

Individual Risk Factors

The risk of getting a disease is related to a number of factors, including genetic predisposition, lifestyle, and occupational exposure [33]. In the United States and other countries, the image of the commercial driver has been perpetuated as the "urban cowboy," roaming free in the great outdoors. Unfortunately, this healthy lifestyle image is not accurate. In a survey of 526 drivers screened with preplacement examinations by Dr. Tuenis Zondag (personal communication) between May 1995 and February 1996, the following general risk factors were noted:

1. Drivers were predominately male (9:1).

2. More than 53 percent of the applicants were more than 30 percent over their ideal body weight.

3. More than 43 percent smoked tobacco.

4. About 12 percent were hypertensive.

5. About 4 percent were diabetic.

6. About 3.5 percent had previous cardiac events.

7. About 14 percent had previous orthopedic injuries.

Males use preventive health services especially infrequently. The individual performing driver examinations has an opportunity to encourage and sometimes demand proactive health attention from a driver to achieve the goal of ensuring public health and welfare and ensuring that the driver "has the ability to drive safely."

An enforcement emphasis project, "Operation Trucker Check," attempted to determine the extent to which commercial tractor-trailer drivers were operating their vehicles while impaired by drugs. Twenty-one percent of the urine specimens tested positive for illicit, prescription, and/or over-the-counter drugs, and 7 percent tested positive for more than one drug. Excluding caffeine and nicotine, the largest number of positive findings (9.5 percent) were for central nervous system stimulants such as methamphetamine, amphetamine, phentermine, ephedrine/pseudoephedrine, and cocaine; 4.3 percent of drivers tested positive for marijuana metabolites; 1.3 percent were positive for alcohol; and 1.6 percent were charged with driving under the influence of drugs after a full Drug Recognition Expert (DRE) evaluation was conducted. Although the drug use is present, only a few drivers were deemed to be under the influence of drugs at the time of driving when evaluated by DRE officers [34].

In a study surveying 2945 male drivers and 353 female drivers done at a trade show for truckers, 54% of male truck drivers smoked cigarettes (versus 30 percent of U.S. white males), 92 percent did not exercise regularly, 50 percent were overweight (versus 25 percent of U.S. white males), and 66% were not aware that they had high blood pressure (versus 46 percent of the U.S. population). Of the surveyed truck drivers, 23 percent tested positive on one measure of alcoholism [35].

To assess the impact of alcohol and other drug use in the trucking industry, the National Transportation Safety Board, in collaboration with the National Institute on Drug Abuse, investigated fatal-to-the-driver trucking accidents in eight states over a 1-year period. Comprehensive drug screens were performed on blood specimens collected from 168 fatally injured drivers. One or more drugs were detected in 67 percent of the drivers, and 33 percent of the drivers had detectable blood concentrations of psychoactive drugs or alcohol. The most prevalent drugs were cannabinoids and ethanol, each found in 13 percent of the drivers. Cocaine or benzoyl ecgonine was found in 8 percent of the cases. Seven percent of the drivers' blood specimens contained amphetamine or methamphetamine, and 7 percent contained phenylpropanolamine, ephedrine, or pseudoephedrine. A panel of toxicologists reviewed the accident investigation report and the toxicology findings for each case and determined that impairment due to marijuana use was a factor in all cases where the delta-9-tetrahydrocannabinol concentration exceeded 1.0 ng/mL and that alcohol impairment contributed to all accidents where the blood alcohol concentration was 0.04% wt./vol. or greater. In 50 of 56 cases where psychoactive drugs or alcohol were found, impairment due to substance use contributed to the fatal accident [36].

Diseases

Many diseases found in commercial drivers mirror the national statistics. However, the prevalence of cardiovascular and musculoskeletal disorders, cancer, diabetes, and sleep disturbances in drivers may be higher than the national average. Excessive daytime sleepiness is related to a significantly higher automotive accident rate in long-haul commercial truck drivers. Sleep-disordered breathing with hypoxemia and obesity are risk factors for automotive accidents. Truck drivers identified with sleep-disordered breathing had a twofold higher accident rate per mile than drivers without sleep-disordered breathing. Accident frequency was not dependent on the severity of the sleep-related breathing disorder. Obese drivers with a body mass index ≥ 30 kg/m^2 also presented a twofold higher accident rate than nonobese drivers [37].

The approach to each disease category will be discussed in the individual chapters. Diabetic drivers of the straight-truck permit class have more accidents than comparable drivers in good health [38]. Occupational hazards, such as general vibration or sitting posture, may result in vertebral neurologic disorders. The location and clinical manifestations of the dysfunction seemed to depend on the intensity and site of action of the hazard [39]. Among commercial drivers, prevalence of back pain due to an injury while working is 6.7 percent [40]. A fourfold increase in the frequency of herniated disk and functional spondyloarthropathies has been found in commercial drivers. Disease of the cervical and lumbar segments also is particularly high [23].

Case-control studies of lung cancer deaths in the Teamsters Union suggest that diesel truck drivers have an excess risk of lung cancer compared with teamsters in positions not in the trucking industry [41,42]. The risk of renal cell carcinoma was found to be associated with employment as a commercial driver or exposure to gasoline, other hydrocarbons, insecticides, or herbicides [43]. Tumors of the lower urinary tract were found to be more common in commercial drivers [44,45]. Males who are normally employed as commercial drivers or deliverymen have a statistically significant 50 percent increased risk of bladder cancer; this trend increases with the duration of commercial driving. Commercial drivers employed 25 years or more show a 120 percent increased risk [46]. Increased mortality for lung cancer and multiple myeloma has been related to diesel exhaust [47]. Commercial drivers of oil tanks showed significantly elevated mortality due to leukemia [48].

One in six heavy-truck drivers and material movers had a diagnosis of alcoholism in a study by Mandell and colleagues [49]. Job dimensions associated with cardiovascular disability were (1) hazardous situations, (2) vigilant work and responsibility for others, (3) exchanging job-related information, and (4) attention to devices [50].

Of 388 drivers screened for sleep apnea, 16 percent were hypertensive, 12 percent of these without previous treatment. Hypertensive drivers were significantly more overweight, slept more restlessly, took more naps, and woke up more frequently during the night. Symptoms indicating regular sleep disturbances were presented by 20 percent of drivers. Long-haul drivers have very irregular sleep/wake schedules and a high prevalence of sleep apnea; this may have an impact on daytime alertness [51,52].

Improving Driver Health

Although it has been long noted that the commercial driver is often not in optimal health, few studies have been done to examine this issue or address methods to improve driver health. In 1997 a Core Wellness Program for drivers was developed and piloted by a consortium of private, government, and industry organizations [53]. Some interesting data in the pretest survey showed

1. Major health concerns of drivers were lack of family time, lack of exercise, weight, fatigue, poor diet, and stress.

2. Drivers were in stages ready or trying to improve behavior in eating, exercise, stress management, self-care, and sleep.

3. Drivers most concerned about health were long-haul drivers 40 to 60 years old and those who did not currently exercise or eat well.

4. Drivers who felt they were in control or were responsible for their own health tended to have better lifestyle habits (i.e., lower weight, more exercise, healthier eating, no tobacco).

After the program, physical improvement measures showing statistical significance were body mass index (from obese as a group to overweight), pulse, diastolic blood pressure, aerobic fitness level (the most improved), strength fitness level, and flexibility fitness level. The program itself had a 96 percent satisfaction rate, with 100 percent recommending the program to others.

The intention of the government and private sectors to actively address the underlying health of this critical workforce is the most noteworthy outcome of such a small study. This is a small step, but an important one.

Conclusion

The process of providing CDL examinations is currently in a state of flux. The principal responsibility of the examiner, regardless of any changes, must still be to protect the public welfare by ensuring that the driver has the "ability to drive safely." Other duties include addressing potential diseases and reviewing current medical conditions. The examiner should give the driver goals and deadlines for complying with measures required to pass the examination. Except for those medical conditions specifically mentioned in the regulation, there are few hard and fast rules to guide the examiner. An understanding of accepted medical practice and good medical judgment remain the basis upon which decisions should be reached.

References

1. U.S. DOT FMCSA, 1999 Safety fitness fact sheet. *http://www.fmcsa.dot.gov/factsfigs/factsheet.htm.* Accessed Jan. 9, 2003.
2. Belkic K, Savic C, Theoreil T, Rakic L, Ercegovac D, Djordejevic M. Mechanisms of cardiac risk among professional drivers. *Scand J Work Environ Health* 1994;20:73–86.

3. Professional Truck Driver Institute. Skill standards for entry-level tractor-trailer drivers. *http://www.ptdi.org/standards/entry_level/ entry02.htm.* Accessed Jan. 8, 2003.

4. Bureau of Labor Statistics. Census of fatal occupational injuries summary. *http://www.bls.gov/news.release/cfoi.nr0.htm.* Accessed Jan. 14, 2003.

5. Bureau of Labor Statistics. Workplace injury and illness summary— 2001. *http://www.bls.gov/news.release/osh.nr0.htm.* Accessed Jan. 14, 2003.

6. Tower W. The hard road: Why the odds are stacked against truckers. *The Washington Post Magazine,* Aug. 5, 2001:11.

7. Apparies R, Riniolo T, Porges S. A psychophysiological investigation of the effects of driving longer-combination vehicles. *Ergonomics* 1998;41(5):581–592.

8. Metzner JL, Tucker GJ, Black DW, et al. *Conference on Psychiatric Disorders and Commercial Drivers.* Publication No. FHWA-MC-01-006. Washington: U.S. DOT, Federal Highway Administration, 1991.

9. Bernard T, Bouck L, Young W. Stress factors experienced by female commercial drivers in the transportation industry. *http:// www.cdc.gov/niosh/elcosh/docs/d0300/d000391/d000391.html.* Accessed Jan. 8, 2003.

10. Mitler MM, Miller JC, Lipsitz JJ, Walsh JK, Wylie CD. The sleep of long-haul truck drivers. *N Engl J Med* 1997;337:755–761.

11. Stoynev A, Minkova N. Circadian rhythms of arterial pressure, heart rate and oral temperature in truck drivers. *Occup Med Oxf* 1997;47(3):151–154.

12. Beilock R. Schedule-induced hours-of-service and speed limit violations among tractor-trailer drivers. *Accid Anal Prev* 1995;27(1):33–42.

13. National Highway Traffic Safety Administration. *The NHTSA & NCSDR Program to Combat Drowsy Driving Report to the House and Senate Appropriations Committee.* DOT HS #808707, April 1998. *http://www.nhtsa.dot.gov/people/perform/human/drowsy2/drdrvrep.htm.* Accessed Jan. 14, 2003.

14. National Highway Traffic Safety Administration. *National Survey for Speeding and Other Unsafe Driving Actions, Volume II: Driver Attitudes & Behavior.* Conducted by Schulman, Ronca & Bucuvalas Inc., Sept. 15, 1998. *http://www.nhtsa.dot.gov/people/injury/aggressive/ unsafe/att-beh/cov-toc.html.* Accessed Jan. 14, 2003.

15. Effects of sleep schedules on commercial motor vehicle driver performance. *http://www.fmcsa.dot.gov/safetyprogs/research/ researchpubs.htm.* Accessed Jan. 8, 2002.

16. Hertz RP. Hours of service violations among tractor-trailer drivers. *Accid Anal Prev* 1991;23:29–36.

17. Moore-Ede MC, Czeisler CA, Richarson GS. Circadian timekeeping in health and disease, 1: Basic properties of circadian pacemaker. *N Engl J Med* 1983;309:469–476.

18. Moore-Ede MC, Czeisler CA, Richarson GS. Circadian timekeeping in health and disease, 2: Clinical implications of circadian rhythmicity. *N Engl J Med* 1983;309:530–536.

19. Stratford D, Ellerbrock TV, Akins JK, Hall HL. Highway cowboys, old hands, and Christian truckers: Risk behavior for human immunodeficiency virus infection among long-haul truckers in Florida. *Soc Sci Med* 2000;50(5):737–749.

20. Burdorf A, Swuste P. The effect of seat suspension on exposure to whole-body vibration of professional drivers. *Ann Occup Hyg* 1993;37:45–55.

21. Piazzi A, Bollino G, Mattioli S. Spinal pathology in self-employed truck drivers. *Med Lav* 1991;82:122–130.

22. Johanning E. Evaluation and management of occupational low back disorders. *Am J Ind Med* 2000;37:94–111.

23. Magnusson M, Pope M, Wilder D, Areskoug B. Are occupational drivers at an increased risk for developing musculoskeletal disorders? Including commentary by King A. *Spine* 1996;21(6):710–717.

24. Casali JG, Robinson GS, Lee SE. *Role of Driver Hearing in Commercial Motor Vehicle Operation: An Evaluation of the FHWA Hearing Requirement.* FHWA PB98-14606. Washington: FHWA, 1998.

25. NIOSH American Conference of Governmental Industrial Hygienists. *Heat Stress: Threshold Limit Values for Chemical Substances and Physical Agents in the Work Environment and Biological Exposure Indices with Intended Changes for 1994.* Cincinnati: American Conference of Governmental Industrial Hygienists, 1995.

26. Steenland K, Deddens J, Stayner L. Diesel exhaust and lung cancer in the trucking industry: Exposure-response analyses and risk assessment. *Am J Ind Med* 1998;34(3):220–228.

27. Hansen ES. A follow-up study on the mortality of truck drivers. *Am J Ind Med* 1993;23(5):811–821.

28. Wong O, Morgan RW, Kheifetws L, et al. Mortality among members of a heavy construction equipment operators union with potential exposure to diesel exhaust emissions. *Br J Ind Med* 1985;42:435–448.

29. Bofetta P, Stellman SD, Garfinkel L. Diesel exhaust exposure and mortality among males in the American Cancer Society prospective study. *Am J Ind Med* 1988;14:403–415.

30. *Health Assessment Document for Diesel Exhaust.* USEPA EPA/600/8-90/057F. 01. Washington: U.S. Environmental Protection Agency, May 2002.

31. Cuddihy RG, McClellan RO, Griffith WC. Potential health risks from increased use of diesel light duty vehicles. *Dev Toxicol Environ Sci* 1982;10:353–367.
32. Belkic K, Savic C, Theoreil T, Rakic L, Ercegovac D, Djordejevic M. Mechanisms of cardiac risk among professional drivers. *Scand J Work Environ Health* 1994;20:73–86.
33. Peterson KW. Disease management: Population-based health management. In: Todd WE, Nash D, eds. *Disease Management: A Systems Approach to Improving Patient Outcomes.* Chicago: American Hospital Publication, 1997:315.
34. Couper FJ, Pemberton M, Jarvis A, Hughes M, Logan BK. Prevalence of drug use in commercial tractor-trailer drivers. *J Forensic Sci* 2002;47(3):562–567.
35. Korelitz JJ, Fernandez AA, Uyeda VJ, Spivey GH, Browdy BL, Schmidt RT. Health habits and risk factors among truck drivers visiting a health booth during a trucker trade show. *Am J Health Promotion* 1993;8(2):117–123.
36. Crouch DJ, Birky MM, Gust SW, et al. The prevalence of drugs and alcohol in fatally injured truck drivers. *J Forensic Sci* 1993;38(6):1342–1353.
37. Stoohs RA, Guilleminault C, Itoi A, Dement WC. Traffic accidents in commercial long-haul truck drivers: The influence of sleep-disordered breathing and obesity. *Sleep* 1994;17(7):619–623.
38. Dionne G, Desjarding D, Laberge-Nadeau C, Maaz U. Medical conditions, risk exposure, and truck drivers accidents: An analysis with count data regression models. *Accid Anal Prev* 1995;27:295–305.
39. Lagutina GN, Tarasova LA, Suvorov GA, Shardakova EF. Effect of work conditions on the development of vertebral neurologic disorders. *Med Tr Prom Ekol* 1994;10:3–6.
40. Behrens L, Seligman P, Cameron L, et al. The prevalence of back pain, hand discomfort and dermatitis in the U.S. working population. *Am J Public Health* 1994;84:1780–1785.
41. Steenland NK, Silverman DT, Hornung RW. Case-control study of lung cancer and truck driving in the Teamsters Union. *Am J Public Health* 1990;80:670–674.
42. *Health Assessment Document for Diesel Exhaust.* USEPA EPA/600/8-90/057F. 01. Washington U.S. Environmental Protection Agency, May 2002.
43. Mellemgaard A, Engholm G, MaLaughlin JK, Olsen JH. Occupational risk factors for renal-cell carcinoma in Denmark. *Scand J Work Environ Health* 1994;20:160–165.

44. Kunze E, Chang-Claude J, Frentzel-Beyme R. Etiology, pathogenesis and epidemiology of urothelial tumors. *Verh Dtsch Ges Pathol* 1993;77:147–156.
45. Boffetta P, Silverman D. A meta-analysis of bladder cancer and diesel exhaust exposure. *Epidemiology* 2001;12(1):125–130.
46. Siverman DT, Hoover RN, Mason TJ, Swanson GM. Motor exhaust-related occupations and bladder cancer. *Cancer Res* 1986;46:2113–2116.
47. Hansen ES. A follow-up study on the mortality of truck drivers. *Am J Ind Med* 1993;23:811–821.
48. Schnatter AR, Katz AM, Nicolich JM, Theriault G. A retrospective mortality study among Canadian petroleum marketing and distribution workers. *Environ Health Perspect* 1993;101:85–99.
49. Mandell W, Eathon WW, Anthony JC, Garrison R. Alcoholism and occupations: A review and analysis of 104 occupations. *Alcohol Clin Exp Res* 1992;16:734–746.
50. Murphy LR. Job dimensions associated with severe disability due to cardiovascular disease. *J Clin Epidemiol* 1991;44:155–166.
51. Stoohs RA, Bingham LA, Itoi A, et al. Sleep and sleep-disordered breathing in commercial long-haul truck drivers. *Chest* 1995;107:1275–1282.
52. Wylie CD, Shultz T, Miller JC, et al. *Commercial Motor Vehicle Driver Fatigue and Alertness Study.* Washington: U.S. Department of Transportation, 1996.
53. Roberts S, York J. *Design Development and Evaluation of Driver Wellness Programs, DOT Technical Memorandum #3.* Washington: DOT, Oct. 31, 1999.

Additional References

Hansson JE. An ergonomic checklist for industrial trucks. In: Zenz C, ed. *Occupational Medicine.* St. Louis: Year Book Medical Publishers, 1988:971–983.

LaDou J. The health of truck drivers. In: Zenz C, ed. *Occupational Medicine.* St. Louis: Year Book Medical Publishers, 1988:958–971.

Pommerenke F, Hegmann K, Hartenbaum NP. DOT examinations: Practical aspects and regulatory review. *Am Fam Phys* 1998;58(2):415–426.

Wells JL, Ferreira DC. Guidelines for the Department of Transportation physical examination. *Nurse Pract* 1999;24(5):78, 81, 88–92.

Index